Dear MyCopy Customer,

This Springer book is a monochrome print version of the eBook to which your library gives you access via SpringerLink. It is available to you at a subsidized price since your library subscribes to at least one Springer eBook subject collection.

Please note that MyCopy books are only offered to library patrons with access to at least one Springer eBook subject collection. MyCopy books are strictly for individual use only.

You may cite this book by referencing the bibliographic data and/or the DOI (Digital Object Identifier) found in the front matter. This book is an exact but monochrome copy of the print version of the eBook on SpringerLink.

V. Bulyzhenkov Y. Christen L. Prilipko (Eds.)

Genetic Approaches in the Prevention of Mental Disorders

Proceedings of the joint-meeting organized by the World Health Organization and the Fondation Ipsen in Paris, May 29–30, 1989

Springer-Verlag Berlin Heidelberg GmbH

Bulyzhenkov, Victor, Dr.
Hereditory Diseases Programme, World Health Organization
Avenue Appia
CH-1211 Geneva 27

Christen, Yves, Dr.
Fondation IPSEN pour la Recherche Therapeutique
30, rue Cambronne
F-75737 Paris Cedex

Prilipko, Leonid, Dr.
Senior Medical Officer
Division of Mental Health, World Health Organization
Avenue Appia
CH-1211 Geneva 27

DOI 10.1007/978-3-662-07421-3

Originally published by Springer-Verlag Berlin Heidelberg New York in 1990.
MyCopy version of the original edition 1990

2127/3140/543210 – Printed on acid-free paper
www.springer.com/mycopy

Preface

At least 40 million people in the world suffer from the most severe forms of mental disorder such as schizophrenia and some 300 million more are affected by less severe but still incapacitating forms of these conditions, including, for example, drug and alcohol dependence and the consequences of brain trauma. The enormous magnitude of human suffering and the economic losses usually linked of these disorders make them a problem of major public health importance.

Recent years have brought with them scientific discoveries which have made it possible to successfully treat most mental disorders and to prevent many others. Some of them, however, cannot be prevented on the basis of today's knowledge, and their treatment remains palliative: further progress in their management awaits an improvement in our understanding of mechanisms by which they come into existence and of factors which influence their course.

Recent years have also seen a significant increase in knowledge about genetic factors influencing the occurrence and course of a variety of diseases, for example, cystic fibrosis, Duchenne type muscular dystrophy, thalassemia, and hypertension. Some of this knowledge and some of the methods that have been developed to obtain it could have direct relevance to the search for a clearer comprehension of the pathogenesis of mental disorder.

At the same time, progress has also been made in relation to the genetics of several mental disorders, for example, Alzheimer's disease, schizophrenia, and manic depressive illness. There is no doubt about the possible usefulness that the factors, methods, and models that have been produced in the genetic research on these disorders could have for the genetics of disease in general.

In order to take these developments into account in its mental health programme, the World Health Organization, in collaboration with the IPSEN Foundation conducted a critical review of knowledge about the genetics of mental disorders, about methods of genetic research into disorders such as schizophrenia and affective psychoses, about their epidemiology, and about issues arising in genetic research. The papers produced on the basis of this review were presented during a meeting which brought together geneticists, epidemiologists, psychiatrists and experts in public health and health ethics. The discussions during this meeting were used in a further revision of the papers, which are here presented to the scientific community, in the hope that they will stimulate the exchange of information and further progress of knowledge about the genetics of mental disorder, of disease in general, and of human development in the absence of disease.

Although the papers included in this volume have been produced in the framework of WHO's review of knowledge about the genetics of mental disorders, they express the views of the individual authors rather than a consensus of the participants at the meeting. Also, the views do not necessarily represent the decisions or stated policy of the World Health Organization or the IPSEN Foundation.

The editors wish to express their appreciation to Mr. G. Dafour, President of the IPSEN Foundation, and Dr. N. Sartorius, Director of the Division of Mental Health, World Health Organization, for their participation in the meaningful discussions during the meeting, and also to Mrs. J. Mervaillie for her assistance in the organization of the meeting and Mrs. M.-L. Gage for her editorial assistance.

V. Bulyzhenkov
Y. Christen
L. Prilipko

Contents

Contributors

Agarwal, S. S.
Sanjay Gandhi Post-Graduate Institute of Medical Sciences,
P.B. 375, Lucknow 226 001, India

Bates, G.
Department of Genome Analysis, ICRF, Lincoln's Inn Fields,
London WC2A, 3PX, UK

Bertelsen, A.
WHO Collaborating Centre for Research and Training in Mental Health,
Institute of Psychiatric Demography, Arhus University Psychiatric Hospital,
DK-8240 Risskov, Denmark

Binková, B.
Psychiatric Research Institute, 181 03 Prague 8, Czechoslovakia

Bloom, F. E.
Research Institute of Scripps Clinic, 10666 North Torrey Pines Road, La Jolla,
CA 92037, USA

Clerget-Darpoux, F.
INSERM U. 155, Château de Longchamp, Bois de Boulogne, F-75016 Paris,
France

Gebhart, J. A.
Psychiatric Research Institute, 181 03 Prague 8, Czechoslovakia

Gill, M.
Institute of Psychiatry, Denmark Hill, London SE5 8AF, UK

Goate, A. M.
Department of Molecular Genetics, St. Mary's Hospital Medical School,
Imperial College London, London W2 1PG, UK

Gottesman, I. I.
Department of Psychology, Gilmer Hall, University of Virginia,
Charlottesville, VA 22904, USA

Lehrach, H.
Department of Genome Analysis, ICRF, Lincoln's Inn Fields,
London
WC2A 3PX, UK

McGue, M.
Department of Psychology, University of Minnesota, 75 East River Road,
Minneapolis, MN 55455, USA

Mendlewicz, J.
Erasme Hospital, Free University of Brussels. Department of Psychiatry,
Route de Lennik 808, 1070 Brussels, Belgium

Murray, R. M.
Institute of Psychiatry, Denmark Hill, London SE5 8AF, UK

Potkin, S.
Department of Psychiatry, University of California, Irvine, CA, USA

Sethi, B. B.
Department of Psychiatry, King George's Medical College, Lucknow, India

Smith, M.
Division of Human Genetics, Department of Pediatrics,
University of California, Irvine, CA, USA

Šrám, R. J.
Psychiatric Research Institute, 181 03 Prague 8, Czechoslovakia

Wertz, D. C.
Boston University School, Health Services Section, 80 East Concord Street,
Boston, MA 02118–2394, USA

Williamson, R.
Department of Molecular Genetics, St. Mary's Hospital Medical School,
Imperial College London, London W2 1PG, UK

Diagnosis and Classification of Mental Disorders in Relation to Molecular Research

A. Bertelsen

Introduction

Accurate and, if possible, correct diagnosis is important in genetic and epidemiological research for obtaining valid estimates of morbid risks in relatives and in the background population for evaluation of heritability and modes of transmission. In molecular genetics diagnosis is of critical importance. In linkage studies just a few misdiagnoses in the pedigrees may ruin the lod scores and prevent the demonstration of linkage and the detection of the gene itself.

In psychiatry diagnostic classification is impeded by nosological difficulties. Only organic disorders approximate nosological entities with known etiology, pathogenesis, symptomatology, and prognosis. The majority of psychiatric disorders are nosographic entities only, syndromes which may overlap, with courses and outcomes which may be more or less characteristic. Etiology is mostly hypothetical, based on competing biological, social and psychological theories. This also applies to the two major groups of disorders, the schizophrenias and the affective disorders. Since their nosographic delimitation by Kraepelin, a genetic etiology has been suspected. Initiated by the Rüdin Institute of Genetic Research, Munich, family, twin and adoption studies have provided increasing evidence of strong genetic factors, but have also shown that genetic factors, if necessary, are not sufficient for the occurrence of the disorders. Other and exogenic factors may enhance or prevent the genetic factors in causing illness. Only the phenotypes, not the genotypes, are available for classification and research. This lack of full expressivity or incomplete penetrance is one of the major obstacles to diagnostic classification as well as to genetic research. The occurrence of phenocopies, nongenetic cases with a clinical appearance similar to the genetic forms, is another obstacle. Organic disorders, for instance, may present themselves with schizophrenic or affective syndromes, such as in Huntington's chorea. Genetic pleiotropy or variable expressivity is a further obstacle, meaning that a genotype may express itself in a number of clinical patterns: for affective disorders not only in manic, depressive and mixed syndromes, but presumably also in schizo-affective disorder and affective personality disorder, and possibly in panic disorder, obsessive-compulsive disorder, and eating disorders. Heterogeneity is still another obstacle, with more than one, maybe many different genes on various locations expressing themselves in the very same syndrome. Recent linkage studies have demonstrated that more than two genes are involved in affective disorders, and more than one in schizophrenia. Correct diagnosis, meaning etiological diagnosis, is therefore difficult to reach. Instead, an accurate clinical diagnosis can be obtained by use of consistent rules of classification and reliable diagnostic criteria.

Diagnostic Criteria for Research

Major contributions to the present classifications of psychiatric disorders came from the German Psychiatric School early in this century. Kraepelin (1909–1915) provided extensive clinical descriptions and an empirically derived classification based on symptoms, course and outcome. Kurt Schneider (1950) later described first-rank symptoms (FRS) of schizophrenia which, in the absence of organic disorder, were considered highly characteristic of schizophrenia. A hierarchy of classification was supposed, with organic psychiatric disorders, schizophrenia, affective disorders, paranoid states, other nonorganic psychoses, and neurotic disorders, and finally personality abnormalities. This hierarchy has been maintained in the World Health Organization (WHO) International Classification of Diseases (ICD) with minor changes through all revisions, of which the ninth is currently in use (World Health Organization 1978). The eighth revision introduced a glossary with brief descriptive diagnostic guidelines allowing a high degree of flexibility and national adaptation at the cost of reliability. The low reliability of diagnostic assessment based on clinical judgment in accordance with varying practices has impeded the comparability of studies, particularly in epidemiological and genetic research. To promote communication between investigators, a number of sets of operationally defined diagnostic criteria have been introduced for more consistent and precise diagnostic assessment, such as the St. Louis criteria (Feighner et al. 1972) and the Research Diagnostic Criteria (RDC) (Spitzer et al. 1975, 1978). They have both had a heavy influence on the American Psychiatric Association Diagnostic and Statistical Manual (DSM) third edition, (DSM-III, American Psychiatric Association 1980) and its latest revision (DSM-III-R, American Psychiatric Association 1987), introducing criteria-based, more accurate diagnostic assessments, also for daily clinical use. The now prefinal draft of the WHO ICD tenth revision has been influenced by the DSM-III versions, with detailed clinical descriptions and criteria-like guidelines in the edition for general use (World Health Organization 1988), and more strictly defined diagnostic criteria in a special edition for research use, the ICD-10-RC (World Health Organization 1989).

The general structure of these classifications includes a number of conditions to be fulfilled for a definite or probable diagnosis. They may require the presence of a basic symptom and a certain number of a variety of accompanying symptoms considered characteristic for the diagnosis. A certain duration and severity may be required and, lastly, one or more exclusion criteria must be observed. For example, for affective disorders disturbed mood is the basic symptom required in all sets of criteria. Four or five of a total of seven or eight accompanying symptoms have to be present with some variation as to extent and degree of severity between the various sets. Duration required for depression varies between 1 month and 1 week; for mania between 2 weeks and 2 days. DSM-III-R has no duration criterion, but instead a severity criterion, demanding hospitalization or markedly impaired occupational or social functioning. The exclusion criteria are more variable, including organic etiology and schizophrenia-like symptoms or illness. The St. Louis criteria have a total of 14 diagnostic groups with two for affective disorders: primary affective disorder, with subdivision into depression and mania, and secondary depression. The RDC has a total of 26 diagnostic groups, of which 12 are affective, including schizoaffective disorders, manic or depressive, and subdivided as to whether they appear mainly affective or schizophrenic. The DSM-III diagnostic criteria include major, other specific, and atypical affective disorders. Manic and major depressive episodes are defined with subtypes of varying severity or specificity, such as melancholia for depression, with and without psychotic symptoms which may be congruent or incongruent with mood, thus allowing the simultaneous presence of schizophrenia-like symptoms. The subgroups include bipolar disorder, mixed, manic or depressed; major depression, single episode or recurrent; cyclothymic and dysthymic disorder; atypical bipolar disorder, and atypical depression. Affective syndromes appear in other categories as organic affective syndrome, schizoaffective disorder (illdefined), and adjustment disorder with depressed mood. The DSM-III-R has rearranged the category of affective disorders, which are now called mood disorders, with manic and major depressive episodes as in DSM-III, with similar subtypes plus a subtype for seasonal pattern of depression. Bipolar disorders now include cyclothymia, and depressive disorders include dysthymia. Outside the category of mood disorders, schizoaffective disorder has been more clearly delineated.

The ICD-10 drafts (World Health Organization 1988, 1989) have followed the DSM-III and DSM-III-R to a high degree with the introduction of nontheoretical operation criteria for research and criteria-like guidelines for general use. For many disorders the criteria closely resemble the DSM- III-R criteria, but there also appear to be major differences and incongruencies. The ICD-10 is the result of the work of many collaborating investigators from all over the world, and it has to be acceptable in a large variety of settings and various psychiatric schools. The ICD-10 for clinical use has to be a sort of "lowest common multiple" of psychiatric disorders and classifications, and therefore cannot be in full accord with any single classification like the DSM-III-R, however desirable this would appear. ICD-10 also tries to assemble affective disorders in a main category of mood disorders, F 3, with subcategories like F 30 – single manic episode – and F-32 – single depressive episode – both with subtypes as to severity and presence of psychotic symptoms, congruent or incongruent with mood, allowing some schizophreniform symptoms to be present. Mild and moderate depression is subdivided as to the presence of melancholiform symptoms which have been named somatic symptoms, although some of the criteria are not so. F 31 includes bipolar disorders and F 33 includes recurrent depressive disorders, both with subtypes as to nature of current episode. F 34 includes persistent affective disorders with cyclothymia and dysthymia. Finally, F 38 and 39 have other and unspecified affective disorders. Originally the F 3 category also included the schizoaffective disorders, which have now been moved to the F 2 category of schizophrenic, schizotypal, and delusional disorders, also including a variety of acute and transient psychotic disorders. Outside the F 3 category affective syndromes appear in F 0: organic disorders and in F 1: disorders due to use of psychoactive substances. F 2 includes, besides the schizoaffective disorders, postschizophrenic depression. Depressive disorders or states are further seen in F 4: mixed anxiety and depressive disorder and adjustment disorder with depressive reaction. The mainly Scandinavian concept of reactive depression and excitation has disappeared into the F 30, 32, and 33 categories, depressive neuroses into F 34 dysthymic disorder, and affective personality disorder into F 34 cyclothymia and dysthymia, and it does not appear in the F 60 subcategory with personality disorders.

The advantage of the use of operational criteria for diagnostic classification is the high reliability of diagnostic assessment which may be obtained. The reliability has been tested for the various sets of criteria, and particularly for the RDC, the DSM-III, and DSM-III-R criteria, high or fairly high reliability coefficients have been obtained for schizophrenia and major affective disorders by both joint and test-retest assessments (Spitzer et al. 1978; American Psychiatric Association 1980, 1987). The coefficients for subtypes of affective disorder are lower, but still satisfactory for research use. For the ICD-10 draft for clinical use, preliminary results have shown satisfactory reliability coefficients for the main categories.

Unsatifactory reliability may, apart from human error, be caused by varying interpretation of the criteria to be used. Furthermore the application of the criteria to diagnostic information involves a clinical judgment open to subjectivity. Even if reliability in a group of investigators is high this is no guarantee of accordance with other groups of investigators using the same classification criteria (Zimmerman 1988).

One of the shortcomings of operational criteria is that they are constrained to the area of definable symptoms. They leave out less definable symptoms like autism, and do not take into consideration the relative weight of individual symptoms or information from keypersons, the personality of the patient, developmental history, interpersonal relationships, or social and cultural background, which may all be decisive for the interpretation of the symptoms and for the clinical diagnosis. The clinical judgment may, therefore, be at variance with the criteria-based evaluation, which might create the temptation to apply the criteria so as to fit the evaluation to the clinical diagnosis. Instead of relying on highly structured interviews with lay-interviewers, and computer techniques for evaluation to compensate for this difficulty, clinical diagnostic evaluation should be considered an indispensable part of the total assessment. Criteria-based evaluation is not "the truth," but an aid to reliable evaluation, and rules for managing cases of disagreement between clinical and criteria evaluation should be established.

Another limitation of the use of operational criteria for classification is the application, in a "top-down" approach, of a rigid set of diagnostic rules, which individual subjects may fail to fulfill. A number of subjects may just fall outside one of the diagnostic categories and have to be categorized in residual, atypical, or unspecified groups, or as "undiagnosed," in spite of an obvious clinical diagnosis. This may be avoided by the use of a different, "bottom-up" way of classification, provided in the "Catego" system in relation to the Present State Examination (Wing et al. 1974). Identified symptoms are grouped into syndromes. The syndromes are further grouped into descriptive categories, which finally converge into one of nine Catego classes, roughly corresponding to major diagnostic groups. The Catego classification is more flexible and also more exhaustive, following hierarchical rules, and the categories and syndromes will thus contain information about symptoms for subjects with less perfect symptom presentation which might otherwise fall short of the "top-down" diagnostic approach.

A further problem in the use of operational criteria is that the discriminatory effect of an inherent hierarchy is partially lost. Although the use of exclusion criteria still present a sort of hierarchy, the authors of DSM-III-R have stated their intention of eliminating previous hierarchies. This will allow subjects to fulfill criteria for more than one diagnostic class. Consequently, subjects who fulfill criteria for, e.g., major depression may simultaneously fulfill criteria for obsessive-compulsive disorder or panic disorder. No rules of diagnostic primacy exist in DSM-III-R, and it is left to clinical judgment whether it is a case of comorbidity of two or more independent disorders, or one major disorder which expresses itself simultaneously in more than one syndrome.

A major criticism of the classifications by operational criteria is their questionable validity. Although high reliability is necessary for establishing validity, it is not sufficient. Various modes of validation have been suggested (Robins and Guze 1970), such as laboratory studies, follow-up studies of course and outcome, and family studies, which have all contributed to the sets of classification criteria and their revisions. All the same, the lack of knowledge of the fundamental etiology makes the operational criteria classifications hypothetical. No single classification set can claim priority, and any set may be applied, although with varying results. In this case it may be advisable to use a polydiagnostic approach (Katschnig and Berner 1983). Multiple sets of criteria may be applied to the subject investigated, for instance by use of the Operational Criteria Checklist for Psychotic Illness (McGuffin and Farmer 1988), for which a computer program provides the diagnostic classifications as to the various sets.

For genetic research the utility of the various classifications may be tried out by applying them in classical research strategies such as twin studies to see which classification produces the most meaningful results. Applied to the Maudsley schizophrenic twin sample, the St. Louis, RDC, and DSM-III criteria all identified as schizophrenic a substantial number of the affected twins (McGuffin et al. 1987). They also produced almost equal concordance rates and ratios and heritability coefficients of the same size. A Schneider's FRS classification identified a low number of cases and was unable to demonstrate any heritability. This may be due to the retrospective character of the application to case record material from interviews, not specifically aimed at detecting Schneiderian symptoms. It is, however, also possible that the symptoms are too infrequent and too specific, at the cost of diagnostic sensitivity, to be useful in genetic research. The ICD-10-RC for schizophrenia relies quite heavily on Schneiderian symptoms and further requires a duration of 1 month. It is thus considerably more strict than DSM-III and DSM-III-R for this disorder.

The usefulness of the various classifications is also seen in their ability to handle the classification of mixed and atypical states, e.g. disorders showing both affective and schizophrenia-like symptoms, either simultaneously or at different times, and maybe in different episodes. In the St. Louis criteria such disorders are classified as "undiagnosed psychotic disorder," except in cases of depression following a schizophrenic syndrome, which is classified as schizophrenia with secondary depression. The RDC is more helpful with two diagnostic groups of schizoaffective disorders, manic and depressed, defined by temporal overlap of active signs of schizophrenia and a full affective syndrome. Each group has four subtypes divided by acute or chronic course and by whether they appear mainly schizophrenic or affective as to primacy and predominance of symptoms and as to premorbid functioning. The RDC schizophrenia diagnosis does not allow simultaneous appearance of prominent affective symptoms, and the manic and major depression disorders have exclusion criteria for schizophrenia-like symptoms. Although of unknown validity, the criteria for RDC schizoaffective disorders have been found quite useful for symptomatological classification in genetic research.

In DSM-III the concept of schizoaffective disorder was considered confusing and controversial and the category was placed in the category of psychotic disorders not elsewhere classified, without delimiting criteria and as a residual for cases which were indiagnosable by the criteria for affective disorders, or schizophrenia and schizophreniform disorder. On the other hand, particularly the criteria for manic and major depression allowed the simultaneous occurrence of mood-incongruent symptoms including FRS, and likewise the criteria for schizophrenia and schizophreniform disorder allowed a full affective syndrome to be present if it developed after the schizophrenic symptoms or was of brief duration. The DSM-III revision, although still stating the doubtful utility of the concept, provided diagnostic criteria requiring both simultaneous occurrence of schizophrenic symptoms and a full affective syndrome, and the appearance of hallucinations or delusions for 2 weeks or more in the absence of prominent mood symptoms, with schizophrenia and organic etiology as exclusion criteria. The criteria for schizophrenia now requires exclusion of schizoaffective disorder, but the criteria for affective syndromes are essentially unchanged.

The ICD-10-RC presents a more strict delimitation of schizoaffective disorders with manic, moderate and severe depressed, and mixed subtypes. Simultaneous and equal or "balanced" occurrence of a full affective syndrome and of one or two of six highly schizophrenia-like symptoms are required. On the other hand, criteria for schizophrenia allow the appearance of an affective syndrome after the development of the schizophrenic disorder, and the affective syndrome criteria allow mood-incongruent psychotic symptoms, except hallucinations and delusions of first-rank character or of pervasive and persistent nature. The various criteria for the schizoaffective disorders are thus not concordant, and it is as yet impossible to state which of the diagnostic systems will prove to be most useful for molecular research. Again, a polydiagnostic approach seems to be the best advice.

Other affective disorders of mixed or atypical character would be mild or moderate depressive syndromes with panic, generalized anxiety, obsessive-compulsive, or somatoform syndromes. The various diagnostic categories provide criteria for the components, giving priority to depression in cases of simultaneous occurrence. For DSM-III and ICD-10 dysthymic disorder criteria, the utility for genetic research still appears undecided. The distinction between endogenous and reactive depression, widely used in Scandinavian psychiatry, has been questioned (Farmer and McGuffin 1989). The criteria for melancholiform subtype of depression in DSM-III and ICD-10 provide a possiblity for further investigations of this problem.

Instruments for Assessment of Mental State in Genetic Research

The assessment of the past and present mental state is a prerequisite for evaluation of lifetime diagnosis by application of the various criteria for classification. It is based on the ascertainment of psychopathology symptoms and signs in probands and their relatives. Information may be obtained from clinical interviews, from medical records, and from relatives with key knowledge of the subjects. Two approaches may be followed: the family study and the family history method. The study method is based on interviews of as many relatives as possible, which is the preferred method in molecular genetic research, where DNA material also has to be obtained. In the family history method information is obtained about all relatives from the proband and one or more key relatives. The history method leads to underreporting, which may be minimized by application of a modification of the research diagnostic criteria: the Family History Research Diagnostic Criteria (FH-RDC) with less rigorous requirements for the less specific information (Andreasen et al. 1977, 1986).

The family history method is more comprehensive because it includes all, even the unavailable, relatives; it is more cheaply and quickly administered and may serve as a screening instrument for detecting informative families. It may also supplement the interview method with otherwise unavailable information about relatives who have moved away or are deceased, or relatives who refuse interview or withhold information. A comparison of the two methods has shown that the family history method has a modest diagnostic sensitivity, but a high specificity which stresses its usefulness as a screening instrument in linkage studies (Thompson et al. 1982).

For the interview a number of instruments have been designed for reliable ascertainment of past and present symptomatology in a standardized and more orless structured way. They consist of questionnaires or rating schedules which may be highly structured with fixed formulations to be used by lay-interviewers, like the Diagnostic Interview Schedule (DIS; Robins et al. 1981) and the Composite International Diagnostic Interview (CIDI; Robins et al. 1988). Less structured and more like a clinical interview, with evaluation by more experienced mental health professionals, are the Schedule for Affective Disorders and Schizophrenia – Lifetime Version (SADS-L; Spitzer and Endicott 1979) and the Structured Clinical Interview for DSM-III (SCID; Spitzer et al. 1988). The Present State Examination, 9th edition (PSE-9; Wing et al. 1974) is semistructured, containing a number of operationally defined psychopathology items which are to be ascertained by an experienced psychiatrist, specially trained for high reliability in using this schedule in accord with a detailed glossary of definitions of symptoms.

The instruments have been developed in relation to the various sets of diagnostic classifications. They contain items and questions to generate information for the criteria to be applied in the corresponding classification for diagnostic assessment. The SADS-L was developed for the RDC. It has a high reliability (Endicott and Spitzer 1978) and has been widely used in genetic research. The SCID was developed for the DSM-III and DSM-III-R classifications and appears quite useful, too. The CIDI is based on the DIS modified for international research, with adopted items from PSE-9. They both generate information for DSM-III, DSM-

III-R, ICD-9 and ICD-10 diagnoses and, by their highly structured design, are most appropriate for use in epidemiological research. The PSE-9 was developed together with the Catego computer classification as a diagnostic reference system reasonably concordant with clinical ICD-9 diagnoses. The PSE-Catego instrument is the most widely used in international clinical and epidemiological research. The PSE covers the last month, but may be extended to any past episodes by a supplementary Past History Schedule (PHS) to produce lifetime evaluations (McGuffin et al. 1986). A 10th edition of the PSE constitutes a nuclear part of a new comprehensive instrument, the Schedules for Clinical Assessment in Neuropsychiatry (SCAN; Wing et al. 1989), capable of generating many of the categories of ICD-10 and DSM-III-R. Preliminary tests indicate reliability similar to that of PSE-9. SCAN was developed under the auspices of WHO-ADAMHA to provide an instrument for international research. The PSE-10 has been expanded by sections not previously included, like cognitive abnormalities, alcohol and substance use, somatoform, dissociative, and eating disorders. Additional schedules collect information about intellectual level, personality disorder, social disablement; information derived from medical records and informants; information on possible causes and pathologies; and supplementary information, mainly about clinical course, relevant to the DSM-III-R and ICD-10 diagnoses. The SCAN covers a variety of present and past periods, including lifetime ever. An expansion of the Catego program is being developed for computer evaluation of Catego classes and diagnoses according to DSM-III-R and ICD-10. The SCAN instrument is being tried in various settings and will be available from 1990.

The instruments used in psychiatric molecular research have so far mostly been the SADS-L in combination with the RDC in full or modified forms, combined with information from hospital records. For affective disorders six linkage studies have recently been published (Baron et al. 1987; Detera-Wadleigh et al. 1987; Egeland et al. 1987; Hodgkinson et al. 1987; Mendlewicz et al. 1987; Gill et al. 1988) and they all used SADS-L and RDC for diagnostic assessment, supplemented by information from medical records and, in two studies, family history information from relatives. Inclusion of diagnostic categories among affected relatives varied from strict bipolar and unipolar affective disorders to schizoaffective and more spectrum-like cases of cyclothymia and anorexia, indicating the variability of expression of the supposed gene. For schizophrenia two recently published studies on linkage to markers on chromosome 5 both used SADS-L and medical records in combination with either RDC and DSM-III criteria or St. Louis and DSM-III criteria (Sherrington et al. 1988; Kennedy et al. 1988).

The recently initiated European Science Foundation Network on Molecular Neurobiology of Mental Illness is trying out both SADS-L and a penultimate draft of the SCAN as instruments for assessment of mental state in probands and affected relatives. For diagnostic evaluation a polydiagnostic approach is planned, including DSM-III-R and ICD-10 criteria (McGuffin and Farmer 1988).

Future Directions and Possible Approaches

Until it becomes possible to detect the endophenotypes, accurate ascertainment of the phenotypes will be a sine qua non in molecular genetics. For homogeneous groups of probands, families informative for linkage studies may be identified by screening with the FH-RDC. In the families selected for study, all available members should be interviewed by a trained and experienced mental health professional supplied with information from medical records and family history information from multiple relatives. The SCAN will probably be preferable to the SADS-L, and the diagnostic assessment will include a clinical diagnosis and a polydiagnostic computer evaluation. The clinical diagnosis tends to be underestimated, but remains indispensable, even if it cannot stand alone. The instruments and diagnostic criteria will need further refinement and inclusion of important, but as yet less definable, symptoms which need further analysis for operational definitions. Information about personality and developmental factors should also be included.

Because the number of highly informative families will be low, international collaboration will be necessary, with the establishment of banks containing pedigrees and DNA material. Molecular genetic research is expensive and will require heavy funding. The rapid evolution of gene mapping techniques, recent discoveries, and the bright prospects for research and treatment have created a strong and positive interest. Detection of closely linked markers will improve diagnostic classification and prediction of risks. Identification of the responsible genes will open up pathogenetic studies, providing insight into the fundamental mechanisms of mental illness. The modes of transmission will become known for the benefit of genetic counseling. The nongenetic factors may be unraveled, opening new possiblities for treatment and prevention. The genetic defects may even finally be accessible to repair.

It is, however, possible that the major mental disorders are heterogeneous and multifactorially determined, as indicated by classical genetics. The preliminary results of the molecular approaches point to heterogeneity in the affective disorders and schizophrenia, and optimism may not be warranted. Anyway, replications and further molecular research are needed before solid knowledge about the etiology of the major psychoses is achieved, and this may still be far ahead.

References

American Psychiatric Association, Committee on Nomenclature and Statistics (1980) Diagnostic and statistical manual of mental disorders, 3rd edn. APA, Washington

American Psychiatric Association (1987) Diagnostic and statistical manual of mental disorders, 3rd edn. revised. APA, Washington

Andreasen NC, Endicott J, Spitzer R, Winokur G (1977) The family history method using diagnostic criteria, reliability and validity. Arch Gen Psychiatry 34:1229–1235

Andreasen NC, Rice J, Endicott J, Reich T, Coryell W (1986) The family history approach to diagnosis. How useful is it? Arch Gen Psychiatry 43:421–429

Baron M, Risch N, Hamburger R, Mandel B, Kushner S, Newman M, Drumer D, Belmaker RH (1987) Genetic linkage between X-chromosome markers and bipolar affective illness. Nature 326:289–292

Detera-Wadleigh SD, Berrettini WD, Goldin LR, Boorman D, Anderson S, Gershon ES (1987) Close linkage of C-Harvey-ras-1 and the insulin gene to affective disorder is ruled out in three North American pedigrees. Nature 325:806–808
Egeland JA, Gerhard DS, Pauls DL, Sussex JN, Kidd KK, Allen CR, Hostetter AM, Housman DE (1987) Bipolar affective disorders linked to DNA markers on chromosome 11. Nature 325:783–787
Endicott J, Spitzer RL (1978) A diagnostic interview, the schedule for affective disorders and schizophrenia. Arch Gen Psychiatry 35:837–844
Farmer A, McGuffin P (1989) The classification of the depressions: contemporary confusion revisited. Br J Psychiatry 155:437–443
Feighner JP, Robins E, Guze SB, Woodroff RA, Winokur G, Munoz R (1972) Diagnostic criteria for use in psychiatric research. Arch Gen Psychiatry 26:57–63
Gill M, McKeon P, Humphries P (1988) Linkage analysis of manic depression in an Irish family using H-ras 1 and INS DNA markers. J Med Genet 25:634–635
Hodgkinson S, Sherrington R, Gurling H, Marchbanks R, Reeders S, Mallet J, McInnis M, Petursson H, Brynjolfsson J (1987) Molecular genetic evidence for heterogeneity in manic depression. Nature 325:805–806
Katschnig H, Berner P (1983) The polydiagnostic approach in psychiatric research. In: World Health Organization: proceedings of the international conference on diagnosis and classification of mental disorders and alcohol and drug related problems. WHO, Geneva
Kennedy JL, Giuffra LA, Moises HW, Cavalli-Sforza LL, Pakstis AJ, Kidd JR, Castiglione CM, Sjøgren B, Wetterberg L, Kidd KK (1988) Evidence against linkage of schizophrenia to markers on chromosome 5 in a northern Swedish pedigree. Nature 336:167–169
Kraepelin E (1909–1915) Psychiatrie, 8th edn. Barth, Leipzig
McGuffin P, Katz R, Aldrich J (1986) Past and present state examination: the assessment of "lifetime ever" psychopathology. Psychol Med 16:461–465
McGuffin P, Farmer AE, Gottesman II (1987) Modern diagnostic criteria and genetic studies of schizophrenia. In: Häfner A, Gattaz WF, Janzarik W (eds) Search for the causes of schizophrenia. Springer, Berlin Heidelberg New York
McGuffin P, Farmer AE (1988) The Operational Criteria checklist for psychotic illness. The European Science Foundation Network on Molecular Neurobiology of Mental Illness
Mendlewicz J, Sevy S, Brocas H, Simon P, Charon F, Legros S, Vassart G (1987) Polymorphic DNA marker on X-chromosome and manic depression. Lancet i:1230–1232
Robins E, Guze SB (1970) Establishment of diagnostic validity in psychiatric illness: its application to schizophrenia. Am J Psychiatry 126:107–111
Robins LN, Helzer JE, Croughan J, Ratcliff KS (1981) National Institute of Mental Health Diagnostic Interview Schedule: its history, characteristics and validity. Arch Gen Psychiatry 38:381–389
Robins LN, Wing J, Wittchen HU, Helzer JE, Babor TF, Burke J, Farmer A, Jablensky A, Pickens R, Regier DA, Sartorius N, Tower LH (1988) The composite international diagnostic interview. Arch Gen Psychiatry 45:1069–1077
Schneider K (1950) Klinische Psychopathologie. 3th edn. Thieme, Stuttgart
Sherrington R, Brynjolfsson J, Petursson H, Potter M, Dudleston K, Barraclough B, Wasmuth J, Dobbs M, Gurling H (1988) Localization of a susceptibility locus for schizophrenia on chromosome 5. Nature 336:164–167
Spitzer RL, Endicott J (1979) Schedule for affective disorders and schizophrenia – lifetime version, 3rd edn. Department of Research Assessment and Training, New York State Psychiatric Institute, New York
Spitzer RL, Endicott J, Robins E (1975) Research diagnostic criteria (RDC). Biometrics Research Department, New York State Psychiatric Institute, New York
Spitzer RL, Endicott J, Robins E (1978) Research diagnostic criteria, rationale and reliability. Arch Gen Psychiatry 35:773–782
Spitzer RL, Williams JBW, Gibbon M, First MB (1988) Structured clinical interview for DSM-III-R – patient version. Biometrics Research Department, New York State Psychiatric Institute, New York
Thompson WD, Orvaschel H, Prusoff BR; Kidd KK (1982) An evaluation of the family history method for ascertaining psychiatric disorders. Arch Gen Psychiatry 39:53–58

Wing JK, Cooper JE, Sartorius N (1974) The measurement and classification of psychiatric symptoms. Cambridge University Press, Cambridge
Wing JK, Babor T, Brugha T, Burke J, Cooper JE, Giel R, Jablensky A, Regier DA, Sartorius N (1989) SCAN: schedules for clinical assessment in neuropsychiatry. Arch Gen Psychiatry (in press)
World Health Organization (1978) Mental disorders: glossary and guide to their classification in accordance with the ninth revision of the international classification of diseases. WHO, Geneva
World Health Organization (1989) ICD-10 1989 draft of chapter V: mental and behavioral disorders, clinical descriptions and diagnostic guidelines. WHO, Division of Mental Health, Geneva
World Health Organization (1989) ICD-10, mental and behavioral disorders, diagnostic criteria for research (April 1989 draft). WHO, Geneva
Zimmermann M (1988) Why are we rushing to publish DSM IV? Arch Gen Psychiatry 45:1135–1138

Genetic Epidemiology Strategies in Psychiatric Diseases

F. Clerget-Darpoux

Summary

In affective disorders and schizophrenia, as in most psychiatric diseases, a genetic component has been shown to exist, but information provided by the segregation of the disease in families is not sufficient to determine the way in which genetic susceptibility is transmitted. To study such diseases with a complex and most likely heterogeneous etiology, genetic epidemiology now focuses on new strategies using genetic markers which can be applied at different levels:

1. At a population level, using "association studies," which compare the marker allele distribution in a sample of unrelated affected individuals with the distribution in a sample of unrelated control individuals.
2. At a family level, using "linkage studies", which test the independence of segregation of the disease and the marker in a family sample.

Results of association and linkage studies must be interpreted with caution, in particular concerning the significance levels attributed and the possible inferences about the etiology of the disease. It is also important to define the population of patients affected by the conclusion. Replication studies are often necessary to obtain good significance levels. The strategy for such replication, as well as possible inferences about the etiology of disease, will be discussed, and an example illustrating the usefulness of genetic markers in the study of complex disorders will be provided, type 1 diabetes.

Introduction

Most psychiatric diseases and, in particular affective disorders and schizophrenia, have been shown to cluster in families. In addition, twin studies, adoption studies, and path analyses have established that at least a part of this family clustering is due to genetic factors (Gottesman 1982, McGuffin and Katz 1989). When there is good evidence for the role of genetic factors, genetic epidemiology aims at finding models of inheritance for genetic susceptibility, and segregation analysis is the most common way of testing a mode of inheritance. In a sample of families segregating the disease, we are confronted with the following question, "Which model best explains the segregation of the disease in these families?"

Three typical modes of segregation are shown in Fig. 1 reproduced from Pellié and Briard (1973):

1. The segregation of a dominant disease with full penetrance, aniridia, where each affected individual has an affected parent.
2. The segregation of a rare recessive disease, Morquio's disease, where parents of the affected individual are unaffected, but where consanguineous mating is often found in the pedigree.
3. The segregation of a recessive sex-linked disease. Duchenne de Boulogne muscular dystrophy, where only males are affected, having inherited the gene for the disease from their mother who is a carrier.

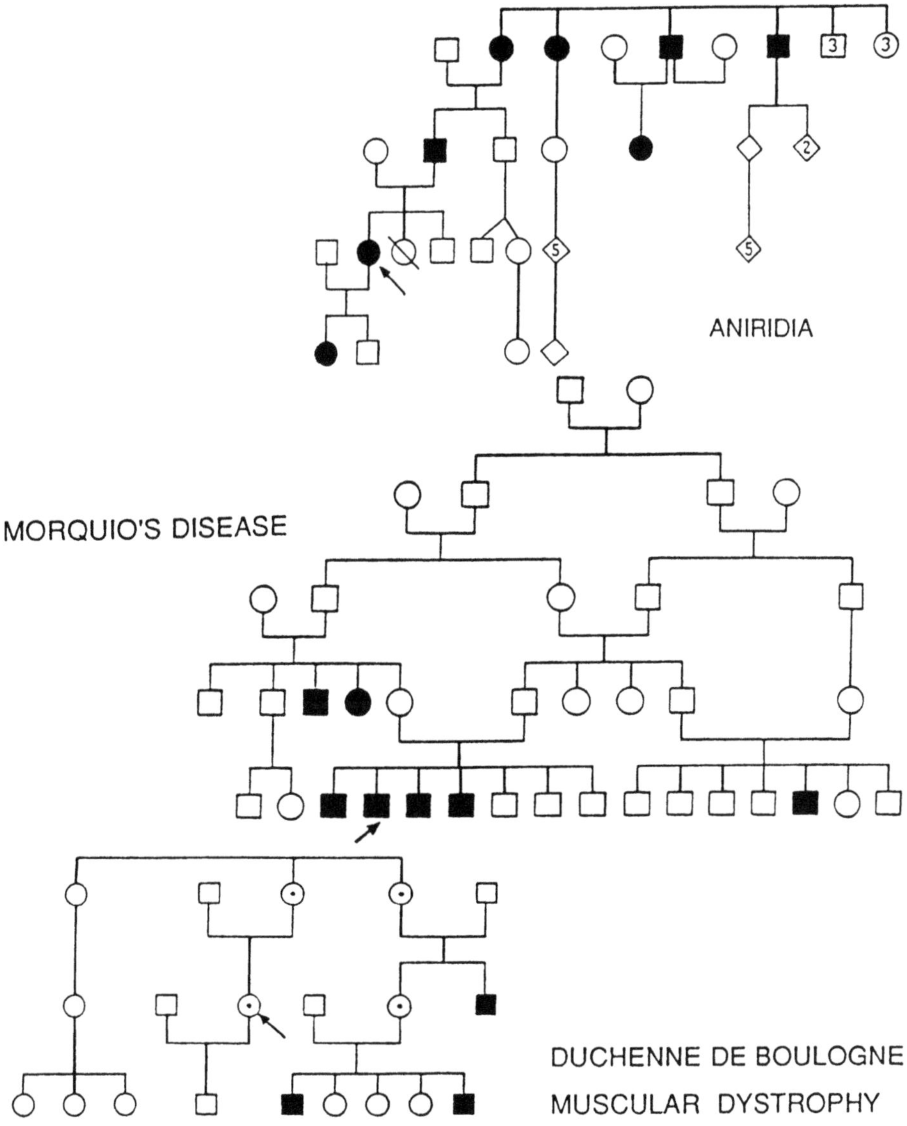

Fig. 1. Three typical modes of segregation

The majority of familial diseases, however, do not follow such a simple mode of transmission, but involve the participation of several factors. When performing a segregation analysis we are in fact asking whether one of the factors involved in the etiology of the disease plays a major role and if it is transmitted in a mendelian manner or, in other terms, is there a "major gene effect"?

For many diseases a genetic component has become evident, but segregation analysis does not reveal the role of a major gene. This is the case for affective disorder and schizophrenia (Goldin et al. 1983; O'Rourke et al. 1982). These disease with complex etiologies are often also likely to be heterogeneous. To study these complex diseases, new strategies are being developed which use the information provided by genetic markers in families of affected individuals.

A genetic marker is a polymorphic gene, i.e., one with multiple allelic forms of expression. The frequencies and dominance relationship of the alleles, as well as the location of the gene on the genome, are known. For example, the ABO blood group system or the HLA system may be considered genetic markers. Thanks to molecular technology, the number of known genetic markers increases very rapidly, and there will soon be markers for any part of the genome. Genetic marker information can be used at a population level by association studies and at a family level by linkage studies.

Association Studies

In an association study between a genetic marker and a disease, the distribution of marker alleles in a sample of unrelated affected individuals is compared with its distribution in a sample of unrelated control individuals. If we consider, for example, a marker with two alleles A_1 and A_2, the contingency table (Table 1) shows the number (expressed by a, b, c, and d) of alleles A_1 and A_2 in samples of both affected and control individuals.

To determine if A_1 is associated with the disease, the frequency of A_1 in affected individuals $a/(a + b)$ is compared with the frequency of A_1 in control individuals $c/(c + d)$. The equality of these frequencies

$$\frac{a}{a+b} = \frac{c}{c+d}$$

is tested using a homogeneity chi-square test with one degree of freedom. If the equality is rejected, association between A_1 and the disease is concluded and a relative risk may be calculated. This risk indicates how many times more fre-

Table 1. Contingency table for testing allociation between the marker allele A_1 and A_2 and a given disease

	A_1	A_2	
Affected	a	b	$a+b$
Control	c	d	$c+d$
	$a+c$	$b+d$	

quently the disease occurs in individuals carrying A_1 versus those not carrying A_1. An approximation of the relative risk (RR) is given by *ad*/*bc*.

Generally, the association test is done not only for one marker and one allele, but for multiple markers with several alleles. In this eventuality, several tests are performed simultaneously on the same sample, and this has to be taken into account when evaluating the significance of the observed differences. Indeed, testing H_0 with a type 1 error $\alpha = 5\%$ means that, when H_0 is correct, one result in 20 (five in 100) is expected to fall outside the confidence limits.

Similarly when performing 20 independent comparisons on one sample, one can expect a difference in one of these comparisons to be significant. A replication study on a different sample is often necessary to attain a good significance level for any given association.

Furthermore, one must be cautious in interpreting an association between a marker allele and a trait. Differences in the distribution of marker alleles may be due to a stratification in the population (noncomplete random mating) that gave origin to the samples. Comparison of frequencies in HLA antigens between dark-haired and blond-haired individuals in Caucasian populations will reveal differences which illustrate a stratification effect.

One possible explanation for an association between a disease and a genetic marker is the existence of a disease susceptibility locus very close to the marker, with a gametic disequilibrium between the marker alleles S_j and the M_i alleles at the disease locus

$$f(M_i S_j) = f(M_i) f(S_j) + \Delta$$

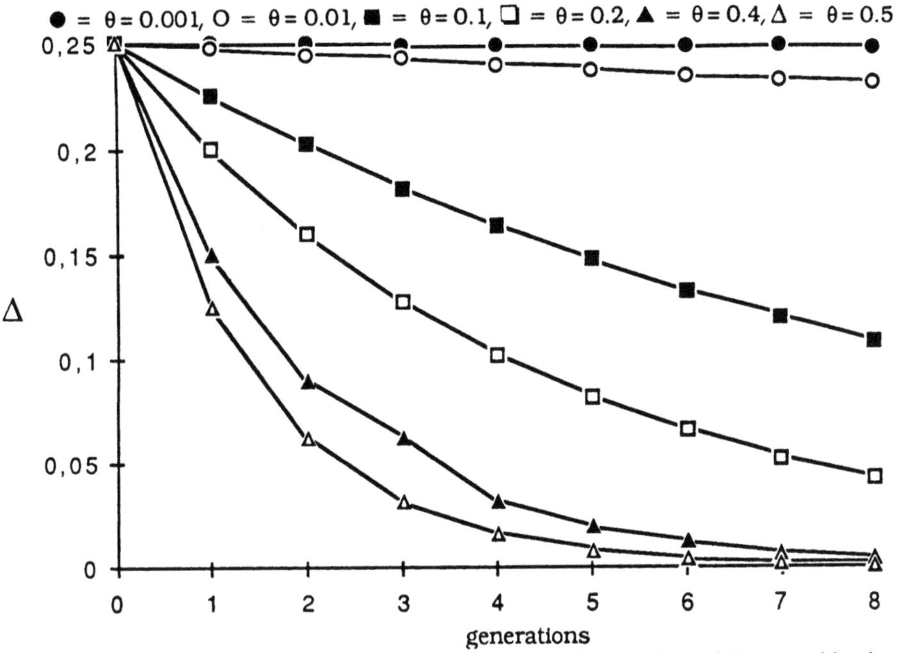

Fig. 2. Decrease of Δ with the number of generations for different values of the recombination fraction θ

Such an explanation has to be confirmed by non-independent segregation in families, as will be explained in the next paragraph.

In the absence of selection or interaction the evolution of a gametic disequilibrium in a panmictic population depends on the recombination fraction between the marker and the disease susceptibility loci. Figure 2 shows the decrease in a given value of Δ with the number of generations for different values of recombination fraction.

Linkage Studies

At the family level a genetic marker can be informative if the disease and the marker do not segregate independently. Illustration of a non-independent segregation of a complex disease and a genetic marker is shown in the pedigree published by Mendlewicz et al. in 1980 (Fig. 3).

In this pedigree we can observe, the segregation of a psychiatric illness – an affective disorder with bipolar and unipolar types – and the segregation of another disease. G6PD deficiency. G6PD may be considered the genetic marker. This gene is located on the X-chromosome and the deficiency is due to a rare recessive allele. Males carrying the deficient allele are affected and carrier females are mothers of affected males. In this pedigree, in nearly all of the individuals over 20 years of age, those having the deficient allele for G6PD have the affective disorder.

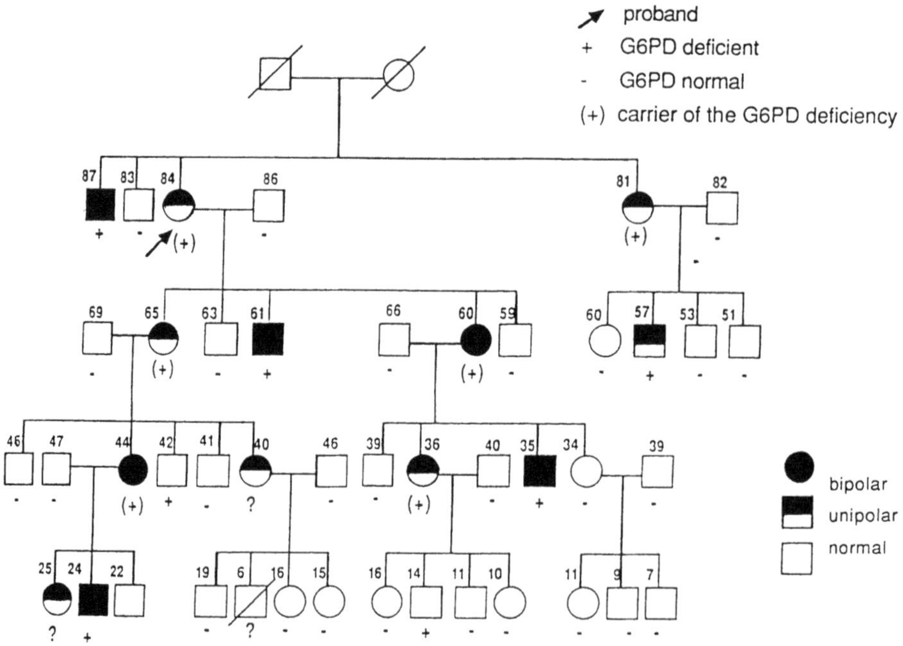

Fig. 3. Co-segregation of affective disorder and G6PD deficiency (Mendlewicz et al. 1980)

A non-independent segregation of a disease and a genetic marker supposes that at least one gene is involved in the etiology of the disease. This gene is necessarily located on the same chromosome pair as the genetic marker at a recombination fraction smaller than 0.50, and eventually is confounded with the marker.

Several methods may be used to test non-independent segregation, including parametric methods requiring disease models, such as the lod score method (Morton 1955), non-parametric methods such as the sib pair method (Penrose 1935) and more extensive methods, such as the affected pedigree member method (Weeks and Lange 1988).

Parametric Method

The most widely used parametric method for testing non-independence or "linkage" is the lod score method. It is not a new approach, since it was first proposed in 1955 by N. Morton. It is important to stress that it was initially developed to locate genes with a known mode of inheritance and not for testing linkage between a complex disease and a genetic marker.

In the usual conditions, i.e., when the disease is monogenic with well-specified genetic parameters (disease allele frequency, dominance relationship between normal and disease alleles, penetrance value), the lod score method can be applied to a sample of families where the segregation of the disease and of a genetic marker is observed. It is then possible to test if the disease and the marker are transmitted independently, i.e., to test the recombination fraction between the disease locus and the marker locus equal to ½, against the linkage at $\theta_1 < ½$, by comparing the likelihoods $L\ (\theta = ½)$ and $L\ (\theta = \theta_1)$. It is equivalent to comparing the probability of observing the data under $\theta = ½$ or $\theta = \theta_1$. For a given family sample, the lod score is defined as

$$Z(\theta_1) = \log_{10} \frac{L(\theta_1)}{L(\theta = ½)}$$

If the lod score $Z\ (\theta_1)$ is greater than or equal to 3, linkage is concluded. The lod score computation, however, is not restricted to a unique value θ_1, but to a set of θ values ranging between 0 and ½. To conclude linkage, the critical value of 3 is than applied to the maximum $Z_{max}\ (\theta)$ of the lod function over the interval [0, ½]. When such a conclusion is reached, the estimate of the recombination fraction is the value which maximizes the lod score function or, equivalently, the value of θ for which the probability to observe the data is maximum. For more details, interested readers may refer to the book edited by J. Ott (1985).

It is impprtant to note that the computations of $L\ (\theta_1)$ and $L\ (\theta = ½)$ and thus of $Z\ (\theta_1)$ are made under certain assumptions and in particular concerning the mode of inheritance of the disease. These assumptions are necessary to infer the probability of genotypes from the observed phenotypes. What happens if these assumptions are incorrect?

We previously studied the effect of different kinds of error in modeling the genetic component of a disease when using the lod score method (Clerget-Darpoux and Bonaiti-Pellie 1980; Clerget-Darpoux 1982; Clerget-Darpoux et al. 1986). More specifically we studied the effect of:

1. Using the wrong genetic parameters for the disease locus (allele frequencies, penetrance values)
2. Ignoring an interaction between the disease locus and the marker locus
3. Ignoring an association between alleles for the disease and the marker loci

We showed that the recombination fraction θ may be very biased when the genetic model is badly specified. For example, underestimating the disease allele frequency q or overestimating the penetrance value f will lead to an overestimation of the recombination fraction θ. Since the disease allele frequency q and the penetrance value f are often constrained by the value of the disease prevalence F in the concerned population, errors in parameters q and f combine to bias the θ estimate. The results of two lod score analyses performed on 52 HLA-typed families with insulin-dependent diabetes, shown in Table 2, illustrate this effect. In both analyses, the disease is assumed to result from a recessive disease allele, but, in the first lod score, $q = 0.065$ and $f = 0.50$, and in the second one, $q = 0.35$ and $f = 0.20$. The location of the disease locus is very different according to the parameter values used. Whereas in the first case the disease locus is far from the HLA marker ($\theta = 0.11$), in the second, when the disease allele is assumed to be very common ($q = 0.35$), the disease locus is within the HLA system ($\theta = 0$).

Table 2. Effect of the genetic parameters on the recombination fraction estimate θ

Disease	Number of families	Parameters		Z_{max}	θ
Insulin-dependent diabetes	52	Recessive	$q = 0.065$ $f = 0.50$	6.83	0.11
		Recessive	$q = 0.35$ $f = 0.20$	7.45	0.00

Let us consider an interaction between the alleles at the marker locus and those at an unlinked disease locus, which is equivalent to assuming a two locus model in which one locus is unlinked and the other is strictly linked to the marker. If the lod score analysis is performed under a one-locus disease model, by ignoring this interaction we would wrongly conclude a loose linkage or, in other words, the existence of a disease locus linked to the marker, but located at a large recombination fraction.

Besides the great sensitivity of the recombination fraction estimation to the genetic modeling of the disease, erroneous modeling can also decrease the maximum lod score (or at least the expected one). This effect is particularly important when a gametic disequilibrium between alleles at the disease and marker loci is ignored. Two consequences can result from this observation. Using the wrong genetic model for the disease may lead to an erroneous rejection of linkage for a given recombination fraction θ, but it does not artificially increase evidence for linkage. This last remark is particularly important with respect to the adequacy of performing a lod score analysis between a disease with an unknown mode of inheritance and a genetic marker. It seems that lod score analysis may be performed if we restrict its use to giving evidence for linkage. This is however true only expectation. It is also important to note that the lod score may be very sensitive to misclassification and that this sensitivity is very dependent on the genetic parameters specified in the linkage analysis.

Nonparametric method

Linkage can also be tested with nonparametric methods such as the sib pair method proposed by Penrose (1935). An extension of this method (Day and Simmons 1976; Thomson and Bodmer 1977; Suarez 1978) has been widely used for testing linkage between the HLA marker and many diseases. The distribution of the number of shared haplotypes in a sample of affected sib pairs is compared with the one expected under independent transmission of the disease and the marker. In the case of the HLA marker, which is highly polymorphic, each parent of a sib pair can be assumed to be HLA heterozygous *(ab)* and different from his or her spouse *(cd)*. In the case for independent transmission of the marker and the disease, if one of the affected sibs is *ac,* the probability for the second sib of sharing 2 HLA haplotypes (i.e., to be *ac*) is ¼, that of sharing one haplotype (*ad* or *bc*) is ½ and that of sharing no haplotypes is ¼. An HLA haplotype shared by two sibs corresponds necessarily to a unique haplotype found in one parent. Two sibs with the same HLA genotype can be considered as identical descent.

On the other hand, if we consider a less polymorphic marker with two alleles, A_1 and A_2, two sibs having A_1 A_2 have not necessarily inherited the same alleles A_1 and A_2. For example, if both parents are A_1 A_2, one of the sibs may have inherited the maternal A_1 and the paternal A_2, but inversely for the second sib. For a less polymorphic marker, the information used is not the identity by descent, but the identity by state. Weeks and Lange (1988) have proposed the use of a variable Z, measuring the degree of identity by state observed between all affected members of a same pedigree. Note that the probability of identity by state for one allele is a function of the probability of identity by descent and of the probability of random identity. For a sample of pedigrees with affected individuals, the observed value of Z may be compared with its value expected with independent segregation.

These parametric and nonparametric approaches each have their advantages and inconveniences. As mentioned above, an erroneous specification of the genetic model in the lod score method decreases the power for detecting linkage. Similarly, the information provided by nonaffected individuals is lost in nonparametric methods. In particular, let us consider two individuals from the same pedigree having the same allele. The probability for this allele to be identical by descent or randomly identical will be computed without considering if intermediate linked individuals in the pedigree have or do not have this allele. Comparisons of the loss of power in different approaches are only possible in specific situations.

Table 3. Reported linkage between markers and complex neuropsychiatric diseases

Affective disorders	Chromosome X (G 6 PD, Xg, colour blindness) (Mendlewicz and Fleiss 1974; Mendlewicz et al. 1980, 1987; Baron 1977; Baron et al. 1987) Chromosome 11 (INS, Hras) (Egeland et al. 1987)
Schizophrenia	Chromosome 5 (D 5 SM 76, D 5 S 39) (Sherrington et al. 1988)
Alzheimer's disease	Chromosome 21 (D 21 S 16) (St. George-Hyslop et al. 1987; Goate et al. 1989)

Illustration

Table 3 shows several examples of linkage between genetic markers and complex neuropsychiatric diseases using a lod score method.

These results must be interpreted with great caution. It is important to note that, when the mode of inheritance of a disease is not perfectly known, it is very tempting to perform lod score analysis using different genetic models or parameter values, different diagnostic criteria for classifying into affected/unaffected individuals, and different genetic markers. We must then deal with the problem of multiple testing since the statistical significance of a maximum lod score greater than 3 is not the same when we perform one or several tests. It is important to perform replication studies using the same genetic model, the same diagnostic classification, and the same genetic marker for which a positive linkage was concluded in the first study.

At present replications of positive findings in psychiatric diseases have not been very encouraging. For affective disorders, Gershon et al. (1979), Leckman et al. (1979), and Kidd et al. (1984) reject linkage with markers of the X-chromosome; Hodgkinson et al. (1987) Detera-Wadleigh et al. (1987) with markers of chromosome 11. For schizophrenia, Kennedy et al. (1988) and St. Clair et al. (1989) reject close linkage with markers of chromosome 5: D5S76, D5S39. Schellenberg et al. (1988) and Pericak-Vance et al. (1988) failed to replicate linkage between Alzheimer's disease and markers of chromosome 21.

Heterogeneity in the etiology of the disease max explain these discrepancies. It emphasizes the importance of comparing the selection criteria of the families studied and of describing the population of patients concerned by the conclusions of a linkage analysis. It would be erroneous to extend the role of a genetic factor evidenced in a given pedigree or family sample to a whole patient population.

Strategies for both replicating a positive finding of linkage and for determining the proportion of patients affected by this linkage are necessary. We considered this question in two studies. In the first one (Clerget-Darpoux et al. 1987) we studied the power to detect heterogeneity in the presence of linkage and the robustness of a homogeneity test, the "admixture test" (Smith 1963), when disease modeling is erroneous. We found the test highly sensitive to the disease modeling when a constraint is fixed on the recombination fraction between the genetic marker and the putative disease locus. However, the use of such constraints may be not only logical if we use a "candidate" gene (potential involvement of this gene in the disease) as a marker, but also necessary if we want to have sufficient power. Using two genetic markers at a known genetic distance will also increase the power of detecting heterogeneity (Lander and Bostein 1986; Martinez and Goldin 1989).

In the second study, Leboyer et al. (submitted for publication) proposed strategies for replication of linkage between affective disorders and markers of chromosomes X and 11. These strategies are proposed for nuclear families assuming different degrees of heterogeneity. It gives the average number of families required to replicate linkage, given the size of the sibship, the number of affected in the sibship, and the parental status for the disease. Both studies show not only the interest of using genetic markers in the region of a candidate gene, but also the caution necessary in interpreting the results.

The usefulness as well as the limitations of genetic marker information in the study of complex disorders are well illustrated by the contribution of the HLA marker to the understanding of type 1 diabetes. Indeed, until recently, it was unclear if different types of diabetes had different etiologies. It is now well established that insulin-dependent diabetes mellitus (IDDM or type 1 diabetes) is associated with an HLA marker and does not segregate independently of this marker in families, but that this is not the case for the other types of diabetes. In Caucasian populations type 1 diabetes is associated with the DR_3 and DR_4 antigens. For example, in a sample of 266 French patients, 95% have either the DR_3 antigen or the DR_4 antigen compared with 32% in a control sample. Moreover, 27% of these patients have the genotype DR_3 DR_4 compared with 3% in the control sample.

Apart from these associations, a non-independent segregation of the HLA marker and type 1 diabetes has also been shown. In a large sample of 185 affected sib pairs 56% are HLA identical, 38% semi-identical and 6% different, which is statistically very different from the 25%, 50%, 25% proportions expected in the case of independent transmission. These well-established observations have been very useful in demonstrating the role of genetic factors located in the HLA region in the etiology of type 1 diabetes. But the exact manner in which these factors and other interacting factors participate in the etiology is still puzzling.

Conclusion

Genetic epidemiology strategies are not the same for diseases with simple modes of inheritance and for diseases with complex modes of inheritance. In the first case, the information provided by the segregation of the disease in families is sufficient to establish the role of a disease gene. The marker information will enable us to locate the disease locus. It may then be possible to determine the defective DNA sequence, and even to determine its activity. For diseases with complex etiology, the trait segregation is not sufficient for inferring the way the susceptibility to the disease is inherited. The additional information provided by genetic markers may be useful in making evident the role of one factor and in subdividing a heterogeneous group of patients into subgroups which are homogeneous for at least one factor. In this way it becomes more realistic to study the role of other potential factors.

Acknowledgments. The author is very grateful to Dr. M. Montès de Oca for editing the English text and to C. Vaillant for typing this manuscript.

References

Baron M (1977) Linkage between an X-chromosome marker (deutan color blindness) and bipolar affective illness. Arch Gen Psychiatry 24:721–727

Baron M, Rish N, Hamburger R et al. (1987) Genetic linkage between X chromosome markers and bipolar affective illness. Nature 326:289–292

Clerget-Darpoux F (1982) Bias of the estimated recombination fraction and lod score due to an association between a disease gene and a marker gene. Ann Hum Genet 46:363–372

Clerget-Darpoux F, Bonaïti-Pellié C (1980) Epistasis effect: an alternative to the hypothesis of linkage disequilibrium in HLA-associated diseases. Ann Hum Genet 44:195–204

Clerget-Darpoux F, Bonaïti-Pellié C, Hochez J (1986) Effects of misspecifying genetic parameters in lod score analysis. Biometrics 42:393–399

Clerget-Darpoux F, Babron MC, Bonaïti C (1987) Power and robustness of the linkage homogeneity test in genetic analysis of common disorders. J Psychiatry Res 21:625–630

Day NE, Simons MJ (1976) Disease susceptibility genes – their identification by multiple case family studies. Tissue Antigens 8:109–119

Detera-Wadleigh SD, Berrettini WH, Goldin L, Boorman D, Anderson S, Gershon ES (1987) Close linkage of C-Harvey-ras and the insulin gene to affective disorders is ruled out in three North American pedigrees. Nature 325:806–808

Egeland JA, Gerhard DS, Pauls DL, Sussex JN, Kidd KK, Allen CR, Hostetter AM, Housman DE (1987) Bipolar affective disorders linked to DNA markers on chromosome 11. Nature 325:783–787

Gershon ES, Targum SD, Matthysse S, Bunney WE (1979) Color blindness not closely linked to bipolar illness. Arch Gen Psychiatry 36:1423–1430

Goate AM, Owen MJ, James LA, Mullan MJ, Rossor MN, Haynes AR, Farral M, Mai LYC, Roques P, Williamson R, Hardy JA (1989) Predisposing locus for Alzheimer's disease on chromosome 21. Lancet I:352–355

Goldin LR, Gershon ES, Targum SD, Sparkes RS, McGinniss M (1983) Segregation and linkage analyses in families of patients with bipolar, unipolar, and schizoaffective mood disorders. Am J Hum Genet 35:274–287

Gottesman II, Shields J, Hanson DR, eds (1982) Schizophrenia. The epigenetic puzzle. Cambridge University. Press Cambridge

Hodgkinson S, Sherrington R, Gurling H, Marchbanks R, Reeders S, Mallet J, McInnis M, Petursson H, Brynjolfsson J (1987) Molecular genetic evidence of heterogeneity in manic depression. Nature 325:805–806

Kennedy JL, Giuffra LA, Moises HW, Cavalli-Sforza LL, Pakstis AJ, Kidd JR, Castiglione CM, Sjøgren B, Wetterberg L, Kidd KK (1988) Evidence against linkage of schizophrenia to markers on chromosome 5 in a northern Swedish pedigree. Nature 336:167–170

Kidd KK, Egeland J, Molthan L, Pauls D, Kruger S, Phil M, Messner K (1984) Amish study. IV. Genetic linkage study of pedigrees of bipolar probands. Am J Psychiatry 141:1042–1048

Lander ES, Botstein D (1986) Strategies for studying heterogeneous genetic traits in humans by using a linkage map of restriction fragment length polymorphisms. Proc Natl Acad Sci USA, 83:7353–7357

Leboyer M, Babron M-C, Clerget-Darpoux F (1989) Sampling strategy in linkage studies of affective disorders. Submitted for publication

Leckman J, Gershon ES, McGinniss MH, Targum SD, Dibble ED (1979) New data do not suggest linkage between the Xg blood group and bipolar illness. Arch Gen Psychiatry 36:1436–1441

Martinez M, Goldin L (1989) The detection of linkage and heterogeneity in nuclear families for complex disorders: one versus two marker loci. Am J Hum Genet, 44:552–559
McGuffin P, Katz R (1989) The genetics of depression and manic-depressive disorder. Br J Psychiatry, pp 155, 294–304
Mendlewicz J, Fleiss JL (1974) Linkage studies with X-chromosome markers in bipolar (manic-depressive) and unipolar depressive illness. J Biol Psychiatry 9:261–294
Mendlewicz J, Linkowski P, Wilmotte J (1980) Linkage between glucose-6-phosphate deshydrogenase deficiency and manic-depressive illness: new evidence. Br J Psychiatry 137:337–342
Mendlewicz J, Simon P, Sevy S, Charon F, Brocas H, Legros S, Vassart G (1987) Polymorphic DNA marker on X chromosome and manic depression. Lancet II:1230–1232
Morton NE (1955) Sequential tests for the detection of linkage. Am J Hum Genet 7:277–318
O'Rourke DH, Gottesman II, Suarez BK, Rice J, Reich T (1982) Refutation of the general single locus model in the aetiology of schizophrenia. Am J Hum Genet 34:630–649
Ott J (1985) Analysis of human genetic linkage. Johns Hopkins University Press, Baltimore
Pellié C and Briard ML (1973) Conseil génétique et hérédité monofactorielle, Revue Pédiatrie, 9:171–178
Penrose LS (1935) The detection of autosomal linkage in data which consist of pairs of brothers and sisters of unspecified parentage. Ann Eugen 6:133–138
Pericak-Vance MA, Yamaoka LH, Haynes CS et al. (1988) Genetic linkage studies in late-onset Alzheimer's disease families. In: Sinet PM, Lamour Y, Christen Y (eds) Genetics and Alzheimer's disease. Springer, Berlin, Heidelberg, New York, pp 116–123
St. Clair D, Blackwood D, Muir W, Baillie D, Hubbard A, Wright A, Evans HJ (1989) Absence of linkage of chromosome 5q11-q13 markers to schizophrenia in Scottish families. Nature 339:305–309
St. George-Hyslop PH, Tanzi RE, Polinsky RJ, Haines JL, Watkins PC, Myers RH, Feldman RG, Pollen D, Drachman D, Growedon J, Bruni A, Foncin JF, Salmon D, Frommelt P, Amaducci L, Sorbi S, Piacentini S, Stewart GD, Hobbs WJ, Conneally PM, Gusella JF (1987) The genetic defect causing familial Alzheimer's disease maps on chromosome 21. Science 235:885–890
Schellenberg GD, Bird TD, Wijsman WM et al. (1988) Absence of linkage of chromosome 21q21 markers to familial Alzheimer's disease. Science 241:1507–1510
Sherrington R, Brynjolfsson J, Petursson H, Potter M, Dudleston K, Barraclough B, Wasmuth J, Dobbs M, Gurling H (1988) Localization of a susceptibility locus for schizophrenia on chromosome 5. Nature 336:164–167
Smith CAB (1963) Testing for heterogeneity of recombination fraction values in human genetics. Ann Hum Genet 27:175–182
Suarez BK (1978) The affected sib pair IBD distribution for HLA-linked disease susceptibility genes. Tissue Antigens 12:87–93
Thomson G, Bodmer W (1977) The genetics of HLA and disease associations. In: Christiansen FB, Fenchel T (eds) Measuring selection in natural populations. Springer, Berlin, Heidelberg, pp 545–564
Weeks DE, Lange K (1988) The affected-pedigree-member method of linkage analysis. Am J Hum Genet 42:315–326

Genetic Linkage in Schizophrenia: Perspectives from Genetic Epidemiology*

M. McGue and *I. I. Gottesman*

Summary

Research on the genetic epidemiology of schizophrenia is briefly and selectively reviewed. Three salient features of schizophrenia that represent challenges to the design of linkage studies are identified. These are:

a) analysis of twin and family data have consistently failed to identify a single major gene effect upon schizophrenia risk;
b) ascertainment of multiplex families does not guarantee the sampling of families who are segregating for the major gene, even if a major gene effect exists, and
c) environmental influences appear to play an essential role in the etiology of at least some schizophrenia. The implications of these features for the design of linkage studies in schizophrenia are discussed.

Introduction

Identifying the genetic mechanisms that underlie individual differences in human behavior remains one of the most significant problems facing the human geneticist. Progress, impeded by the complexity of the behavioral phenotype, has been slow, however. It is little wonder then that the advent of the application of molecular genetic methods to human behavior (Gurling 1986) and the recent successes in linking behavioral conditions, including affective psychoses (Egeland et al. 1987), reading disability (Smith et al. 1983), Alzheimer's disease (St. George-Hyslop et al. 1987), and schizophrenia (Sherrington et al. 1988) to specific regions of the genome have given rise to much optimism. Clearly the race has begun to apply molecular genetic techniques to the study of human behavior. As behavioral geneticists we have long been interested in the way knowledge of a genetic influence will bring about a better understanding of the development of psychopathology with an eye toward rational intervention and even prevention. It appears an especially appropriate time to consider whether behavioral pathology is best treated as other human genetic disorders (i.e., more grist for the human geneticist's mill), or whether the study of genetic influences on behavior will require new and unique research approaches.

* This article is published simultaneously in Schizophrenia Bulletin (1989) 15:281–292

Throughout its development, behavioral genetics has relied heavily upon the biometrical approach, the galtonian paradigm. This approach, although statistically sophisticated, has been widely criticized because of its inability to characterize the mechanisms of genetic influence (e.g., Vogel and Motulsky 1986). Over the past 22 years, we have engaged in biometrical analyses of schizophrenia twin and family data (Gottesman and Shields 1967; Rao et al. 1981; McGue et al. 1983, 1986). Although we agree that these analyses do not allow us to identify the underlying genetic processes, we believe they do help us to understand the genetics of schizophrenia. Indeed, as the field embarks upon intensive molecular genetic studies of schizophrenia, the results of our biometrical analyses may have implications for the probable success of alternative strategies for identifying single gene effects on schizophrenia. We consider those results and some of their implications here.

Genetic Epidemiology of Schizophrenia

The most powerful and consistent predictor of schizophrenia risk is being an identical twin of first-degree relative of a schizophrenic (Gottesman et al. 1982; Eaton 1985). Table 1 gives estimated lifetime risks (i.e., age-corrected values) for developing schizophrenia among the relatives of schizophrenics pooled from systematic studies undertaken in Western Europe since 1920 (for a complete description of how the data were compiled, see Gottesman et al. 1982 and Slater and Cowie 1971). Values for a broader definition, including "probable schizophrenia", are about 25% higher than those given in the table. With the exception of the twin data, where a large correlation in age of onset as well as continued follow-up obviates the need, all risks have been adjusted for variable age of onset using variations of the Weinberg method (Gottesman et al. 1982).

There is a strong association between the magnitude of the risk in the relative and the degree of genetic relationship to the proband. The most distinctive features of this association are the monozygotic (MZ) twin concordance rate and the risk to the offspring of two schizophrenics, both of which are large relative to the risks among other family members. The MZ rate is approximately five times the

Table 1. Rates of definite schizophrenia among the relatives of schizophrenics

Familial relationship	BZN[a]	Percentage affected
Offspring of two schizophrenics	134	36.6
MZ twins	106	44.3
DZ twins	149	12.1
Siblings	7523	7.3
Offspring of one schizophrenic	1678	9.4
Half-siblings	442	2.9
Nieces or nephews	3965	2.7
Grandchildren	739	2.8
First cousins	1600	1.6
Spouses	399	1.0

[a] BZN gives the age-adjusted sample size (Gottesman et al. 1982)

rate among first-degree relatives, which in turn is approximately two and one-half times the rate among second-degree relatives. The association between familial risk and proportion of genes shared with the index case is approximated by an exponential decay function (Fig. 1). Alternative hypotheses about the genetic transmission of schizophrenia are distinguished by their ability to account for this essential epidemiological association.

Twin, adoption, and family studies are consistent in indicating that the familial aggregation of schizophrenia is accounted for largely, if not entirely, by genetic factors (Rosenthal 1972; McGue et al. 1986). Nonetheless, the MZ twin concordance rate is substantially less than 100%, and thus (nonfamilial) environmental factors, be they prenatal, perinatal, or sociocultural, play a significant role in the etiology of at least some forms of schizophrenia. The existence of environmental influences serves to obscure the mechanism of genetic transmission, resulting in continued debate as to whether schizophrenia is a single-gene disorder, multifactorially transmitted, or etiologically heterogeneous (Faraone and Tsuang 1985).

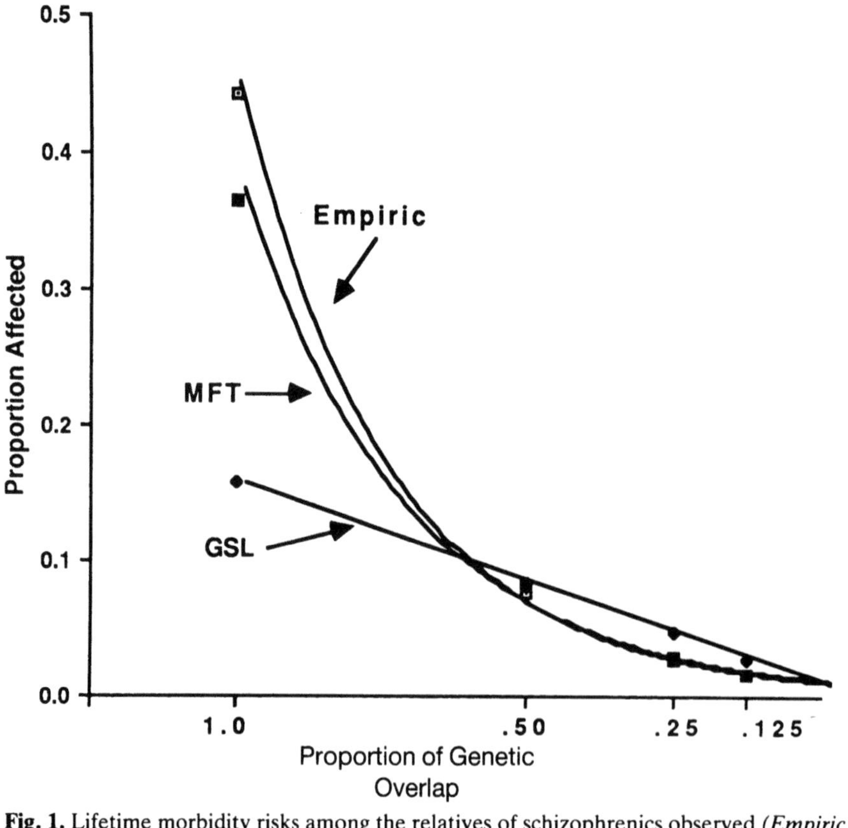

Fig. 1. Lifetime morbidity risks among the relatives of schizophrenics observed *(Empiric)* and expected under a multifactorial threshold model with 80% heritability *(MFT)* and the generalized single-locus model *(GSL)* proposed by Matthysse et al. (1986), as a function of proportion of genes shared with the proband. Proportion of genetic overlaps is 1.0 for MZ twins, 0.50 for first-degree relatives, 0.25 for half-siblings, and 0.125 for third-degree relatives

This is not a purely academic concern, as the likelihood of identifying single-gene effects on schizophrenia risk depends upon the mode of transmission of the disorder.

Single-Gene Transmission

A prominent hypothesis (in fact the first historically, Rosanoff and Orr 1911; Rudin 1916) for the genetic basis of schizophrenia is that it is a single-gene defect (Book 1953; Slater 1958; Heston 1970; Slater and Cowie 1971; Matthysse et al. 1986). Under the so-called generalized single locus (GSL) model, the transmission of schizophrenia is attributed solely to the segregation of two alleles (a schizophrenia-promoting allele, say A, and a non-schizophrenia-promoting allele, say a) at a single locus. Nonmendelian familial risks are reconciled with single gene transmission by invoking reduced penetrance (i.e., individuals who inherit at least one copy of the disease-promoting gene do not necessarily develop the disorder) and allowing for the existence of sporadics (i.e., individuals who inherit no copies of the disease-promoting gene, but who are still at risk). Table 2 gives the parameterization of the GSL model in terms of the frequency of the schizophrenia-promoting allele *(a)* and the penetrances of the three genotypes (f_{AA}, f_{Aa}, and f_{aa}).

Table 2. Parameterization of the generalized single-locus model

Genotype	AA	Aa	aa
Frequency	q^2	$2q(1-q)$	$(1-q)^2$
Penetrance	f_{AA}	f_{Aa}	f_{aa}

Both the parsimony as well as the assumption of a unitary genetic etiology for schizophrenia that promises success for molecular genetic strategies make the GSL model attractive. Nonetheless, the GSL model has repeatedly failed to account for the observed pattern of familial risk in schizophrenia (Elston and Campbell 1970; Kidd and Cavalli-Sforza 1973; Elston et al. 1978; O'Rourke et al. 1982; Tsuang et al. 1982; Baron 1986; McGue et al. 1986). This failure stems from the inability of the GSL model to predict an exponential relationship between familial risk and degree of the relationship with the proband.

James (1971) has shown how precise quantitative predictions of familial risks can be determined under a GSL model. The risk to relatives of a given class K_r can be expressed as a function of three parameters derivable from the penetrances and gene frequency of the GSL model; the population prevalence of the disorder K_p, the additive genetic variance V_a, and the dominance genetic variance V_d;

$$K_r = K_p + (\mu_1 V_a + \mu_2 V_d)/K_p \qquad (1)$$

where μ_1 and μ_2 are the probabilities that the proband and the relative share, respectively, one or two alleles at a locus identical by descent.

In the absence of dominance (as appears to be the case for schizophrenia, where the risk to the siblings is not greater than the risk to the offspring of schizophrenies), predicted familial risk under the GSL model is given by a linear function of proportion of genetic overlap between the relative and the proband. That is, in the absence of dominance, Eq. 1 is reduced to

$$K_r = K_p + (V_a/K_p)\,\mu_I \tag{2}$$

This linear prediction is in sharp contrast to the observed exponential relationship. Along with the empiric risks, Fig. 1 plots the familial risks predicted by a recently proposed, and illustrative, GSL model of schizophrenia (Matthysse et al. 1986). The degree of reduced penetrance required under a GSL model to account for the low familial recurrence of schizophrenia is clearly inconsistent with the relatively large MZ twin concordance rate. In those cases where the GSL model did fit shizophrenia family data, observations were made only on first-, second-, and third-degree relatives, but not twins or the offspring of dual matings (e.g., Holzman et al. 1988). Figure 1 shows that the linear relationship between risk and shared genetic background predicted by the GSL model holds approximately only for these classes of relatives.

Failure of the GSL model leads not only to rejection of simple single-gene explanations for the transmission of schizophrenia, but also to rejection of the hypothesis that schizophrenia represents a heterogeneous mixture of single-gene disorders only. Suppose that there were *k* different single-gene defects, each of which gives rise, with possibly reduced penetrance, to schizophrenia. Neglecting those exceedingly rare cases who inherit more than one of these genes, the composite risk to a relative of a schizophrenic index case is a probability-weighted function of that relative's risk under each of the *k* separate single-gene models. That is, the composite familial risk, being approximated by a weighted average of *k* separate linear functions, will also be a linear function of proportion of genes shared with the proband.

A simple hypothetical example should serve to illustrate. Suppose that the transmission of schizophrenia depended on two separate single-gene defects, either of which alone could produce the disorder. The first is a rare, completely penetrant (i.e., individuals who inherit at least one copy of the gene are affected regardless of status at any other locus) dominant gene with a gene frequency of 0.002. The second is a common, incompletely penetrant gene with a frequency of 0.03 and a penetrance vector of $f_{AA} = 0.20$, $f_{Aa} = 0.10$ and $f_{aa} = 0.002$. Risks generated under such a heterogeneity model are approximately linearly related to degree of genetic relatedness between the proband and the relative. The expected MZ concordance rate is 0.391 (a value not that dissimilar from observed values), but the risk to the offspring of schizophrenics is 0.201 (a value clearly greater than those observed). The failure of simple single-gene models to account for schizophrenia family data complicates the search for single-gene effects. This failure does not exclude the possibility that schizophrenia may, in some cases, be due to a rare, highly penetrant gene effect. Rather it excludes the possibility that schizophrenia is a heterogeneous mixture of single-gene effects.

Multiple-Gene Models

Multiple-gene models do not share the empirical shortcomings of the GSL model. Although many alternative multiple-gene models have been proposed, we will focus upon the two most widely applied, the multifactorial threshold (MFT) and mixed models. Under a MFT model, genetic factors are assumed to be polygenic. That is, there is a large number of genes, each of small and equal effect, that combine additively with the effects of other genes and environmental factors to influence schizophrenia liability. The qualitative phenotype (here a diagnosis of schizophrenia) is assumed to arise when an individual's combined liability exceeds some threshold value along the unobserved liability continuum (Falconer 1965; Gottesman and Shields 1967).

The MFT model does an excellent job in accounting for the distinctive pattern of familial risk in schizophrenia (McGue et al. 1983). Figure 1 gives the predicted rates of schizophrenia under a MFT model that assumes all familial transmission is due to polygenic factors with a multifactorial heritability of 80%, with the remaining 20% of the liability variance being attributed to nonfamilial environmental effects (McGue et al. 1985). Although the predicted MZ concordance rate is somewhat low, this model is statistically consistent with the observed familial rates and, more importantly, produces a risk function with the characteristic exponential decline.

Despite its predictive adequacy, there exists a general reluctance to accept the MFT model as an explanation for the transmission of schizophrenia. This reluctance stems, perhaps, from the failure to identify specific genetic and environmental contributors to the assumed multifactorial liability. Additionally, strict polygenic inheritance (i.e., many genes all of small effect) would likely preclude, for the near future, attempts at identifying single-gene effects on schizophrenia risk through molecular genetic approaches. However, the fit of the MFT model does not preclude the existence of a single major gene whose effect upon schizophrenia risk is large relative to the effects of other (poly)genes, the possibility of rare single-gene disorders that give rise to schizophrenia, or a tractable MFT model of a limited number of polygenes (3, 4 or 5), each with a "subcomponent effect" on schizophrenia (cf. Wright 1934; Thoday 1967). Molecular genetic strategies could, presumably, be tailored for each of the possibilities.

Meehl (1972a, b) was the first to suggest that both a major gene and polygenes play a role in the etiology of schizophrenia. Under Meehl's theory, inheritance of a single gene gives rise to a neural integrative deficit termed schizotaxia that is expressed at the personality level as schizotypy. Expression of clinical schizophrenia among individuals who inherit the single-gene defect is postulated to be a function of status on a host of polygenically and environmentally influenced potentiators, including anxiety, anhedonia, and social introversion.

The type of model proposed by Meehl has been termed the mixed (i.e., mixed major and polygenes) model by the human geneticists Morton and McClean (1974), who also developed analytical procedures for fitting the model to family data. Although the procedures outlined by Morton and McClean can be used, in theory, to identify major gene effects against a polygenic background, in practice, the analysis of qualitative family data under the mixed model has yielded equivocal results. There have been three mixed model analyses of schizophrenia family data (Carter and Chung 1980; Risch and Baron 1984; Vogler et al. 1989). In all three cases, the researchers failed to reject the multifactorial model that included polygenic effects only, in favor of a mixed model that included both a single major gene and polygenic effects. That is, they failed to find support for a single major effect upon schizophrenia risk. This failure may result from a lack of statistical power *or* to an absence of a single major gene effect on schizophrenia. With the given data it is difficult to resolve the choice between these two possibilities, although the repeated failure to identify single major gene effects schizophrenia, despite relatively large family studies, suggests that, if single-gene effects exist, they may be of modest magnitude only.

Simulation Studies

To identify the characteristics of mixed single-gene/polygene models that generate accurate predictions of familial risk, we recently completed a simulation study (Gottesman and McGue 1989). In that study, familial risks under 275 different models were computed and compared with observed schizophrenia risks. Family data were generated under a general model that allowed for three additive contributors to schizophrenia liability:

a) a major gene component with two alleles *A* and *a* at a single locus in Hardy – Weinberg equilibrium;
b) a polygenic component that was assumed to be normally distributed with a constant variance for the three genotypes *AA, Aa,* and *aa;* and
c) a *nonfamilial* environmental component, also assumed to be normally distributed with a constant variance.

Familial environmental effects, for which there is little empirical evidence (McGue et al. 1985), were not modeled in the simulation. The penetrances of the three genotypes were ordered according to $f_{AA} > f_{Aa} > f_{aa}$ with the heterozygote penetrance f_{Aa} constrained to equal the average of the penetrances of the two homozygotes, as is expected when there is no dominance variance at the single locus. In all cases, the lifetime prevalence of schizophrenia was fixed at 1.0%.

Familial risks were functions of three (input) parameters:

a) f_{AA}, the penetrance of the most frequently affected genotype;
b) *s,* the percentage of schizophrenics who do not have any copies of the "schizophrenia gene" (i.e., the proportion of schizophrenics with the *aa* genotype termed the proportion of sporadics; and
c) h^2, the residual polygenic heritability (i.e., the proportion of liability variance due to polygenic factors after the major gene effect has been partialled out).

Table 3 gives illustrative findings from these simulations. Three general conclusions were drawn:

1. When the penetrance of the most frequently affected genotype was high ($f_{AA} \geq 0.4$), predicted familial risks were inconsistent with observed risks unless *both* the percentage of schizophrenics without the major gene was high ($s \geq 0.60$)

and the residual heritability was large ($h^2 \geq 0.60$). Put another way, if there exists a highly penetrant major gene for schizophrenia, simulations of family data suggest that few schizophrenics possess it. This is illustrated in Table 3 by the comparison of the three inconsistent models numbered 5, 6 and 7 with the consistent model numbered 2.
2. When the penetrance of the most frequently affected genotype was low ($f_{AA} \leq 0.2$), predicted familial risks were inconsistent with observed risks unless the residual heritability was large ($h^2 \geq 0.60$). Put another way, a low-penetrant gene is consistent with schizophrenia family data only when there is also a substantial polygenic effect. This is illustrated in Table 3 by the two consistent models numbered 1 and 3 and the two inconsistent models numbered 8 and 9.
3. A pure MFT model with large heritability ($h^2 = 0.80$) yields familial risks consistent with observed risks. This is illustrated by the consistent model numbered 4 in Table 3.

These simulations suggest that three alternative classes of genetic models are consistent with the genetic epidemiology of schizophrenia: first, a heterogeneity-like model where the minority of schizophrenics inherit a highly penetrant, but low frequency gene (gene frequencies for models numbered 1 and 2 were, respectively, 0.003 and 0.018) while the majority are affected because of a high multifactorial loading; second, a gene of modest effect model where a low penetrance (about 10%), moderately prevalent (gene frequency for model 3 was 0.097) gene contributes along with a sizable multifactorial component to schizophrenia risk; and third, a pure MFT model. Any one of these models could account for the failure of mixed model analyses of schizophrenia family data to identify a single major gene effect.

Table 3. Illustrative results from the mixed model simulation of schizophrenia (Gottesman and McGue 1989)

Model	Input parameters			Derived parameters (%) Total variance due to:			Predicted risks to relatives of schizophrenics (%)			
No.	f_{AA}	s	h^2	Major gene	Polygene	Environment	MZ	1st	2nd	3rd
Consistent models										
1	0.10	0.80	0.80	2.2	78.3	19.5	41.3	9.3	3.6	2.0
2	0.60	0.80	0.80	2.3	78.2	19.5	45.1	11.6	4.7	2.6
3	0.10	0.025	0.60	32.9	40.3	27.8	43.6	10.8	4.1	2.2
4	0.0	1.0	0.80	0.0	80.0	20.0	38.3	8.6	3.3	1.9
Inconsistent models										
5	0.60	0.60	0.20	4.9	19.0	76.1	17.1	8.1	4.3	2.6
6	0.60	0.05	0.60	18.9	48.7	32.4	59.2	22.0	9.8	5.0
7	0.60	0.05	0.20	18.9	16.2	64.9	37.8	17.2	8.6	4.7
8	0.10	0.025	0.40	32.9	26.8	40.3	24.9	7.6	3.3	2.0
9	0.10	0.80	0.40	2.2	39.1	58.7	10.5	4.0	2.1	1.5

Abbreviations: f_{AA} penetrance of the most frequently affected genotype; s proportion of schizophrenics who do not carry the major gene; h^2 residual multifactorial heritability

Ascertainment Strategies

The results of our simulations suggest that the existence of a single major gene effect is not inconsistent with the observed schizophrenia family data, although the magnitude of this effect on overall risk may not be great. If a single major gene exists, the question remains as to how best to sample pedigrees of families for linkage studies who are informative with respect to the major gene. One popular, and seemingly sensible, strategy for identifying families for intensive molecular genetic study is to sample "loaded pedigrees" (i.e., so-called multiplex families with a large number of affected individuals). We were interested in determining, for the four models found to generate risk rates consistent with the observed familial rates, the extent to which.

a) families with multiply affected members are expected to occur, and
b) multiplex ascertainment schemes succeed in enriching the sample with families who are segregating for the major gene.

For each of the four models, 50 000 nuclear families consisting of an index member (not necessarily affected) and possibly a spouse (probability of marriage was 0.864) and up to six children were generated according to the parameters of that model. Probability of marriage and number of offspring were chosen to reflect demographic features of the United States adult population. No adjustment was made for the reduction in fertility known to be associated with schizophrenia (Erlenmeyer-Kimling 1978; Vogel 1979; Odegaard 1980). Average number of offspring was 2.22 (SD = 1.4, range = 0–6).

Table 4 gives the distribution of the number of affected individuals among families with at least one affected member. Two features of Table 4 warrant comment. First, all four models predict that, in a large percentage of cases, schizophrenics will be the only affected members of their nuclear family. This prediction is in accord with the distribution of number of affected family members observed in large family studies (e.g., Lindelius 1970). Second, although rare, pedigrees with multiple affected members are expected under all four models of transmission. Although expected under highly penetrant single-gene transmission, the observation, especially under uncertain ascertainment, of loaded pedigrees does not allow unequivocal inference of mode of transmission. Indeed, of the total of

Table 4. Distribution of number of affected nuclear family members under four alternative models for schizophrenia

	Model input parameters[a]			Number (%) of affected members per family				
No.	f_{AA}	s	h^2	1	2	3	4 or more	Total[b]
1	0.10	0.80	0.80	1156 (0.912)	97 (0.076)	14 (0.011)	1 (0.001)	1268
2	0.60	0.80	0.80	1133 (0.909)	99 (0.079)	12 (0.010)	3 (0.002)	1247
3	0.10	0.025	0.60	1311 (0.894)	112 (0.085)	24 (0.018)	3 (0.003)	1311
4	0.0	1.0	0.80	1214 (0.918)	88 (0.067)	17 (0.013)	4 (0.003)	1323

[a] See Table 3 for abbreviations; [b] Total number of nuclear families of the 50 000 generated with at least one schizophrenic member

Table 5. Proportion of schizophrenics without the major gene $P(G^-IS^+)$ and proportion of normals with the major gene $P(G^+/S^-)$ under three alternative ascertainment schemes[a]

Affected familiy members	Model 1 $P(G^-/S^+)$	Model 1 $P(G^+/S^-)$	Model 2 $P(G^-/S^+)$	Model 2 $P(G^+/S^-)$	Model 3 $P(G^-/S^+)$	Model 3 $P(G^+/S^-)$
1 or more	0.748	0.089	0.879	0.035	0.026	0.480
2 or more	0.658	0.089	0.789	0.054	0.000	0.427
3 or more	0.652	0.028	0.542	0.125	0.000	0.516

[a] Less than 25 observations, proportion not calculated

200 000 nuclear families generated, only two contained as many as five affected members. One family was generated under model number 3, a mixed model with high multifactorial heritability, and the other under model number 4, a pure MFT model.

Table 5 gives the sample proportions of

1. affected individuals who carry no copies of the schizophrenia-promoting gene ($P(G^-/S^+)$), and
2. normal individuals who carry at least one copy of the schizophrenia-promoting gene ($P(G^+/S^-)$) under alternative sampling schemes for each of the three models for which there os a major gene effect.

These proportions can be interpreted loosely as error rates under the alternative ascertainment schemes, that is, the chance that an affected individual in the sample does not have the gene and the chance that a normal individual does. As is evident from the table, multiplex sampling strategies do not insure that observed affected family members carry the major gene in those cases where a major gene effect exists. Under models numbered 1 and 2, multiplex sampling had a discernible, but extremely modest effect in reducing the "false-negative" rate. Only for model number 3, where the gene frequency is high, but the penetrance low, are most sampled families expected to be segregating the major gene.

Nonetheless, in this case a significant proportion of unaffected individuals also possess the gene, and this "false-positive" rate is not improved through multiplex sampling.

The Role of the Environment

The existence of environmentally induced schizophrenic-like conditions (Davison 1987) as well as MZ twin concordance rates substantially less than 100% prompts the question: is the influence of the environment on schizophrenia due primarily to environmentally induced phenocopies of the disorder, or is it that environmental effects combine multifactorially with an underlying genetic diathesis? We note that the popular distinction between sporadic and familial forms of psychopathology presumes that a major role of the environment is to induce nontransmitted forms of the disorder (see, however, Eaves et al. 1986 for a critical evaluation of this distinction as applied in genetic epidemiology).

Table 6. Schizophrenia and schizophrenia-like psychosis in offspring of discordant twins (Gottesman and Bertelsen 1989)

Monozygotic sample			
Parent status	Number	Affected[a]	MR (%)[b]
Affected twin	14	1	10.0 ± 9.0
Unaffected twin	24	4	17.4 ± 7.7
Dizygotic Sample			
Parent status	Number	Affected	MR %
Affected Twin	13	1	8.3 ± 7.6
Unaffected Twin	52	1	2.1 ± 2.1

[a] Total number of offspring affected with either schizophrenia or a schizophrenic-like psychosis
[b] Estimated lifetime morbid its risk with the Kaplan Meier age correction procedures

Gottesman and Bertelsen (1989) evaluated schizophrenia risk among the offspring of Fischer's concordant and discordant twins. Relatively low rates of schizophrenia are expected among the offspring of discordant MZ twins if discordance among the genetically identical parents is due largely to environmentally induced phenocopies. Table 6 gives the essential findings from this study. Although the small sample allows only preliminary and cautiously drawn conclusions, the pattern of offspring risk is striking. For the discordant MZ twins, the rate of schizophrenia-like psychosis is similar among the offspring of the affected and the unaffected twins and both rates are comparable to the overall risk to the offspring of a schizophrenic parent (see Table 1). In contrast, for the discordant dizygotic (DZ) twins, the rate of schizophrenia-like psychosis is significantly higher among the offspring of the affected twin than among the offspring of the unaffected twin. Furthermore, the rate among the offspring of the affected DZ twins is comparable to the rate among the offspring of schizophrenics, while the rate among the offspring of the unaffected co-twins is comparable to the risk among the second-degree relatives of schizophrenics (see Table 1).

These data suggest that the discordance among the MZ twins be attributed entirely to the existence of nontransmissible forms of schizophrenia. Apparently, the expression of schizophrenia depended upon both an inherited genetic diathesis, which was transmitted regardless of whether the diathesis was phenotypically expressed, and exposure to environmental stressors, to which the twins are differentially exposed. The possibility that the expression of schizophrenia might depend upon exposure to requisite environmental triggers would seem to complicate, but certainly not preclude, genetic linkage studies which are highly sensitive to the existence of "false-negatives" in the family.

Discussion and Conclusion

Alternative approaches to identifying single major gene effects on schizophrenia will be constrained, encouraged, and/or defeated by salient features of the genetic epidemiology of this complex disorder. Here, we have reviewed three such features, all of which have significant implications for designing linkage studies of schizophrenia. First, nobody has ever been able to demonstrate statistically that a single major gene accounts for a large share of the overall risk for schizophrenia. We suggest that this reflects more about the nature of this complex disorder than it does about limitations in the statistical procedures. Approaches premised upon the hypothesis that schizophrenia is a unitary single-gene disorder run counter to a vast amount of empirical data that suggest otherwise. At the least, such approaches need to be justified relative to their more empirically attractive alternatives.

Single-gene effects on schizophrenia risk may exist. Our simulations suggest that if they do, they are likely to be the result of either a highly prevalent gene with a very low penetrance or a very low prevalent gene with a high penetrance. In either case, the contribution to overall schizophrenia risk is modest. For example, Huntington's disease (HD) is often misdiagnosed as paranoid schizophrenia; some 20% of HD cases present with paranoid schizophrenia phenotypes. HD is quite rare in the population with an incidence of 5 per 100 000. From the careful total population study in southern Sweden by Essen-Moller et al. (1956) that used indepth interviews by psychiatrists with every inhabitant, we obtain a lifetime risk of 139 per 10 000 for schizophrenia. We can now answer the question, what proportion of schizophrenia-like psychoses are actually caused by what we now know to be a mutated dominant gene on chromosome 4 leading to HD? The answer is found by dividing the two population values, or 5/100 000 by 139/10 000, and then taking 20% to get those HD cases who are, in this instance, "genocopies" of schizophrenia. The result of the calculations is that 7 in 10 000 schizophrenics have this "major gene for schizophrenia-like psychosis" and the gene would be identified by studying such special pedigrees with RFLPs (restriction fragment length polymorphisms) and a lucky choice of chromosome 4 as a starting place.

Second, ascertainment schemes aimed *only* at identifying "loaded pedigrees" may be useful, but then again they may not. Obviously, linkage studies require loaded pedigrees to provide powerful test for single-gene effects. Nonetheless, multiplex families are expected under GSL and MFT transmission. This may leave the molecular geneticist somewhat uneasy in claiming that the family he or she is expending great effort on happens to be a family segregating for the major gene. It is notable in this regard that the linkage studies for mental disorder that are currently available, whether for schizophrenia or affective psychoses, were conducted without defining a sampling framework. We have no way of knowing how many families in the general population were, in effect, screened to find the interesting multiplex families utilized to obtain the significant lod score. Under such conditions, the linkage studies resemble the important data available from individual case histories provided by such pioneers as Freud, Kraepelin, and E. Bleuler. As such, pedigrees with impressive lod scores as well as seminal case histories can serve as hypothesis-generating sources, but not as sufficient proof of etiology.

Third, environmental influences play an essential role in the etiology of schizophrenia. In the rush to molecular biology, it would appear short-sighted for psychopathologists to no longer consider why it is that, among two individuals, both of whom inherit a genetic diathesis, one will go on to develop the disorder while the other will not. It would seem that progress will be maximized by tying molecular genetic approaches to further inquiry into environmental influence.

The simulation results, as well a empirical data, suggest that linkage studies of schizophrenia which are fishing expeditions may yield only few successes. An attractive alternative, broadly supported by our research, is the targeted strategy of the candidate gene approach (Gurling 1986). Wright (1934) and Thoday (1967) have shown how a multifactorial system can be broken down into a small and tractable number of single-gene effects (say, 3, 4, or 5). Lander and Botstein (1989) have developed linkage analysis methods which can be used with such systems in experimentally bred species. Appropriate strategies in humans may be forthcoming. Likely sources for candidate genes would be single-gene effects upon the many correlates of schizophrenia, including D_2 dopamine receptors (Wong et al. 1986), cerebral blood flow asssessed with positron emission tomography (Early et al. 1987), cerebral ventricle size (Reveley et al. 1984), and smooth pursuit eye tracking (Iacono et al. 1981; Holzman et al. 1988).

Research on the genetic epidemiology of schizophrenia suggests that is is a highly complex genetic disorder whose precise mechanism of transmission remains uncertain. This will hardly come as a revelation to anyone. The pathway from gene product to be behavioral expression is obviously long and presumably provides many opportunities for environmental modulation as well as moderation by other biological, physiological, and behavioral systems. The transmission of schizophrenia appears completely unlike the transmission of HD and cystic fibrosis. Coronary heart disease and diabetes may represent more appropriate models for designing linkage studies of schizophrenia. The challenge that psychopathology presents to the geneticist is not so much in finding multiplex families that can be intensively studied, but rather in adapting approaches that have proven useful with relatively simple medical genetic disorders to account for the complexities, heterogeneity, and environmental sensitivity of human behavior.

Acknowledgments. This work was supported in part by NIH grant RR01632. We would like to thank Michael Goay for assistance in generating the data used in the simulations.

References

Baron M (1986) Genetics of schizophrenia: I. Familial patterns and mode of inheritance. Biol Psychiatry 21:1051–1066

Book JA (1953) A genetic and neuropsychiatric investigation of a North Swedish population. Acta Genet Stat Med 4:1–100

Carter CL, Chung CS (1980) Segregation analysis of schizophrenia under a mixed model. Hum Hered 30:350–356

Davison K (1987) Organic and toxic concomitants of schizophrenia: association or chance? In: Helmchen H, Henn FA (eds) Biological perspectives of schizophrenia. Wiley, New York, pp 139–160

Early TS, Reiman EM, Raichle ME, Spitznagel EL (1987) Left globus pallidus abnormality in never-medicated patients with schizophrenia. Proc Nat Acad Sci USA 84:561–563

Eaton WW (1985) Epidemiology of schizophrenia. Epidemiol Rev 7:105–126

Eaves LJ, Kendler KS, Schulz SC (1986) The familial sporadic classification: its power for the resolution of genetic and environmental etiologic factors. J Psychiatr Res 20:115–130
Egeland JA, Gerhard DS, Pauls DL, Sussex JN, Kidd KK, Allen CR, Hostetter AM, Housman DE (1987) Bipolar affective disorders linked to DNA markers on chromosome 11. Nature 325:783–787
Elston RC, Campbell MA (1970) Schizophrenia: evidence for a major gene hypothesis. Behav Genet 1:3–10
Elston RC, Namboodiri KK, Spence MA, Rainer JD (1978) A genetic study of schizophrenia pedigrees. II. One-locus hypotheses. Neuropsychobiology 4:193–206
Erlenmeyer-Kimling L (1978) Fertility of psychotics: demography. In: Cancro R (ed) Annual review of the schizophrenic syndrome, vol 5. Brunner Mazel, New York, pp 298–333
Essen-Moller E, Larson H, Uddenberg CE, White G (1956) Individual traits and morbidity in a Swedish rural population. Acta Psychiatr Neurol Scand [Suppl] 100
Falconer DS (1965) The inheritance of liability to certain diseases estimated from the incidence among relatives. Ann Hum Genet 29:51–76
Faraone SV, Tsuang MT (1985) Quantitative models of the genetic transmission of schizophrenia. Psychol Bull 98:41–66
Gottesman II, Bertelsen A (1989) Confirming unexpressed genotypes for schizophrenia: risks in the offspring of Fischer's Danish identical and fraternal discordant twins. Arch Gen Psychiatry (in press)
Gottesman II, McGue M (1989) Mixed and mixed-up models for the transmission of schizophrenia. In: Cichetti D, Grove W (eds) Thinking clearly about psychology: essays in honor of Paul E. Meehl. University of Minnesota Press, Minneapolis (in press)
Gottesman II, Shields J (1967) A polygenic theory of schizophrenia. Proc Natl Acad Sci USA 58:199–205
Gottesman II, Shields J, Hanson DR (1982) Schizophrenia: the epigenetic puzzle. Cambridge, Cambridge Press
Gurling H (1986) Candidate genes and favoured loci: strategies for molecular genetic research into schizophrenia, manic depression, autism, alcoholism and Alzheimer's disease. Psychiatr Dev 4:289–309
Heston LL (1970) The genetics of schizophrenia and schizoid disease. Science 167:249–256
Holzman PS, Kringlen E, Matthysse S, Flanagan SD, Lipton RB, Cramer G, Levin S, Lange K, Levy DL (1988) A single dominant gene can account for eye tracking dysfunctions and schizophrenia in offspring of discordant twins. Arch Gen Psychiatr 45:641–647
Iacono WG, Tuason VB, Johnson RA (1981) Dissociation of smooth pursuit and saccadic eye tracking in remitted schizophrenics. Arch Gen Psychiatr 38:991–996
James JW (1971) Frequency in relatives for an all-or-none trait. Ann Hum Genet 35:47–49
Kidd KK, Cavalli-Sforza LL (1973) An analysis of the genetics of schizophrenia. Soc Biol 20:254–265
Lander ES, Botstein D (1989) Mapping Mendelian factors underlying quantitative traits using RFLP linkage maps. Genetics 121:185–199
Lindelius R (1970) A study of schizophrenia: a clinical prognostic, and family investigation. Acta Psychiatr Scand [Suppl] 216
Matthysse SW, Holzman PS, Lange K (1986) The genetic transmission of schizophrenia: application of mendelian latent structure analysis to eye tracking dysfunctions in schizophrenia and affective disorder. J Psychiatr Res 20:57–65
McGue M, Gottesman II, Rao DC (1983) The transmission of schizophrenia under a multifactorial threshold model. Am J Hum Genet 35:1161–1178
McGue M, Gottesman II, Rao DC (1985) Resolving genetic models for the transmission of schizophrenia. Genet Epidemiol 2:99–110
McGue M, Gottesman II, Rao DC (1986) The analysis of schizophrenia family data. Behav Genet 16:75–87
Meehl PE (1972a) A critical afterword. In: Gottesman II, Shields J (eds) Schizophrenia and genetics, a twin study vantage point. Academic, New York, pp 367–415
Meehl PE (1972b) Specific genetic etiology, psychodynamics, and therapeutic nihilism. Int J Ment Health 1:10–27
Morton NE, MacLean CJ (1974) Analysis of family resemblance. III. Complex segregation analysis of quantitative traits. Am J Hum Genet 26:489–503

Odegaard O (1980) Fertility of psychiatric first admissions in Norway 1936–1975. Acta Psychiatr Scand 62:212–220
O'Rourke DH, Gottesman II, Suarez BK, Rice J, Reich T (1982) Refutation of the general single-locus model for the etiology of schizophrenia. Am J Hum Genet 34:630–649
Rao DC, Morton NE, Gottesman II, Lew R (1981) Path analysis of qualitative data on pairs of relatives: application to schizophrenia. Hum Hered 33:325–333
Reveley AM, Reveley MA, Murray RM (1984) Cerebral ventricular enlargement in nongenetic schizophrenia: a controlled twin study. Br J Psychiatry 144:89–93
Risch N, Baron M (1984) Segregation analysis of schizophrenia and related disorders. Am J Hum Genet 36:1039–1059
Rosanoff AJ, Orr FI (1911) A study in insanity in the light of the Mendelian theory. Am J Insanity 68:221–261
Rosenthal D (1972) Three adoption studies of heredity in the schizophrenic disorders. Int J Ment Health 1:63–75
Rudin E (1916) Zur Vererbung und Neuentstehung der Dementia Praecox. Springer, Berlin
Sherrington R, Brynjolfsson J, Pekursson H, Potter M, Dudleston K, Barraclough B, Wasmuths J, Dobbs M, Gurling H (1988) Localization of a susceptibility locus for schizophrenia in chromosome 5. Nature 326:164–167
Slater E (1958) The monogenetic theory of schizophrenia. Acta Genet Stat Med 8:50–56
Slater E, Cowie V (1971) The genetics of mental disorders, Oxford University Press, London
Smith SD, Kimberling WJ, Pennington BF, Lubs HA (1983) Specific reading disability: identification of an inherited form through linkage analysis. Science 219:1345–1347
St. George-Hyslop PH, Tanzi RE, Polinsky RJ et al. (1987) The genetic defect causing familial Alzheimer's disease maps on chromosome 21. Science 235:885–890
Thoday JM (1967) New insights into continuous variation. In: Crow JF, Neel JV (eds) Proceedings of the 3rd international congress of human genetics. Johns Hopkins, University Press, Baltimore, pp 339–350
Tsuang MT, Bucher KD, Fleming JA (1982) Testing the monogenic theory of schizophrenia: an application of segregation analysis to blind family data. Br J Psychiatry 140:595–599
Vogel F, Motulsky AG (1986) Human genetics: problems and approaches. Springer, Berlin Heidelberg New York
Vogel HP (1979) Fertility and sibship size in a psychiatric patient population: a national comparison with census data. Acta Psychiatr Scand 60:483–503
Vogler GP, Gottesman II, McGue MK, Rao DC (1989) Mixed model segregation analysis in thc Lindelius Swedish pedigrees. Behav Genet (in press)
Wong DF, Wagner HN, Tune LE et al. (1986) Positron emission tomography reveals elevated D_2 dopamine receptors in drug-naive schizophrenics. Science 234:1558–1563
Wright S (1934) An analysis of variability in number of digits in an inbred strain of guinea pigs. Genetics 19:506–536

New Genetic Strategies in Neuropsychiatric Disorders

J. Mendlewicz

Among the various psychoses, major affective illness – in particular, manic-depression – has been the primary subject of many classic genetic studies. Table 1 summarizes concordance rates for manic-depression in twin studies of manic-depressive probands (Mendlewicz 1988). Concordance rates are consistently higher in monozygotic (MZ) than dizygotic pairs, but they do not reach the 100% value in MZ pairs, indicating that nongenetic (environmental) factors may also be operational in this illness, and interacting with the genetic predisposition. Such interactions between nature and nurture can be best examined through the use of more sophisticated strategies, such as the adoption method and the new linkage analyses. The adoption method has been applied to manic-depression with conclusive results (Mendlewicz and Rainer 1977) demonstrating the necessary presence of important genetic factors (Table 2). More recent linkage studies with classic genetic markers such as color blindness and G6PD deficiency have provided consistent evidence of the presence of a major single gene located on the distal end of the long arm of the X-chromosome in bipolar manic-depression (Mendlewicz 1986, 1988), despite the fact that this type of inheritance has not been observed in all families studied (Mendlewicz 1988). In addition, using the DNA recombinant method in molecular genetic studies of manic-depression, a close linkage has recently been demonstrated between manic-depression and factor IX (hemophilia B) on the distal end of the long arm of chromosome X in a new set of pedigrees (Mendlewicz et al. 1987), as illustrated in Fig. 1. Furthermore, the localization of a gene situated on the distal part of the short arm of chromosome 11 has also been reported in one family originating from the old Amish community (Egeland et al.

Table 1. Concordance rates for manic-depressive illness in monozygotic (MZ) and dizygotic (DZ) twins (Mendlewicz 1988)

Study	Concordance rate %	
	MZ	DZ
Rosanoff et al. (1934)	69.9	16.4
Kallmann (1954)	92.6	23.6
Da Fonseca (1959)	71.4	38.5
Harvald and Hauge (1965)	50.0	2.6
Kringlen (1967)	33.3	0.0
Bertelsen (1977)	58.0	17.0
Torgersen (1986)	75.0	0.0

Table 2. Diagnosis of parents for normal adoptees and nonadoptes (Mendlewicz and Rainer 1977)

Adoptive parents	Normal adoptes ($N = 24$)						Poliomyelitis ($N = 20$)		
	Biological parents			Biological parents					
	Male	Female		Male	Female		Male	Female	
Bipolar	0	0	(0)	0	0	(0)	0	0	(0)
Unipolar	1	2	(3)	1	0	(1)	3	1	(4)
Schizoaffective	0	0	(0)	0	0	(0)	0	0	(0)
Cyclothymic	1	0	(1)	0	0	(0)	0	0	(0)
Affective Spectrum	2	2	(4)	1	0	(1)	3	1	(4)
Percentage	10	10	(10)	5	0	(2)	15	5	(10)
Schizophrenia	0	1	(1)	0	0	(0)	0	0	(0)
Alcoholism	0	0	(0)	1	2	(3)	1	0	(1)
Sociopathy	0	0	(0)	2	1	(3)	0	0	(0)
Other	0	0	(0)	0	1	(1)	0	0	(0)
All psychopathology	2	3	(5)	4	4	(8)	4	1	(5)
Percentage	9	14	(11)	18	18	(18)	20	5	(12)

1987), but this chromosomal linkage has not yet been confirmed in other pedigrees (Detera-Wadleigh et al. 1987; Hodginkson et al. 1987; Michael et al. 1988).

Thus, these new chromosomal linkage findings suggest the existence of several distinct genetic forms of bipolar illness, with at least two different chromosomal locations, one on the tip of the long arm of the X-chromosome and the other (if confirmed) on the short arm of chromosome 11, as illustrated in Figs. 2 and 3. Other pedigrees of bipolar illnesses have been reported not to show linkage with these genetic markers (Mendlewicz 1988). These results provide strong support for the hypothesis of molecular heterogeneity in the genetic etiology of bipolar

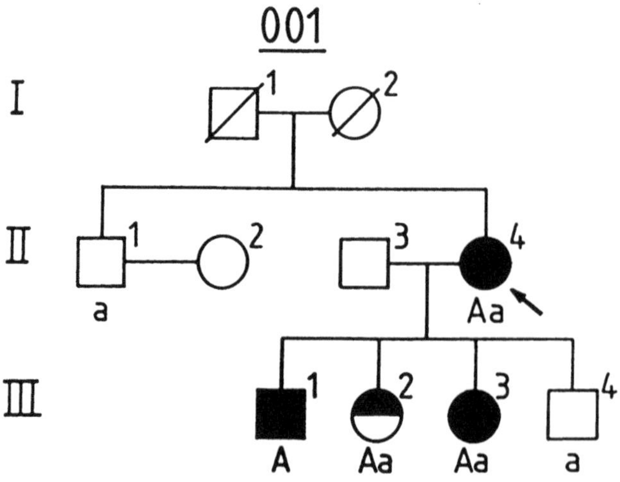

Fig. 1. Pedigree of one family. 0, females; □, males; *black symbol* subject with bipolar (full) or unipolar (half) illness; *slashed symbol*, subject deceased; *arrow*, propositus; *A*, *a*, phenotypes at factor IX locus (*A* allele 1.8 kb, *a* alele 1.3 kb. (From Mendlewicz et al. 1987)

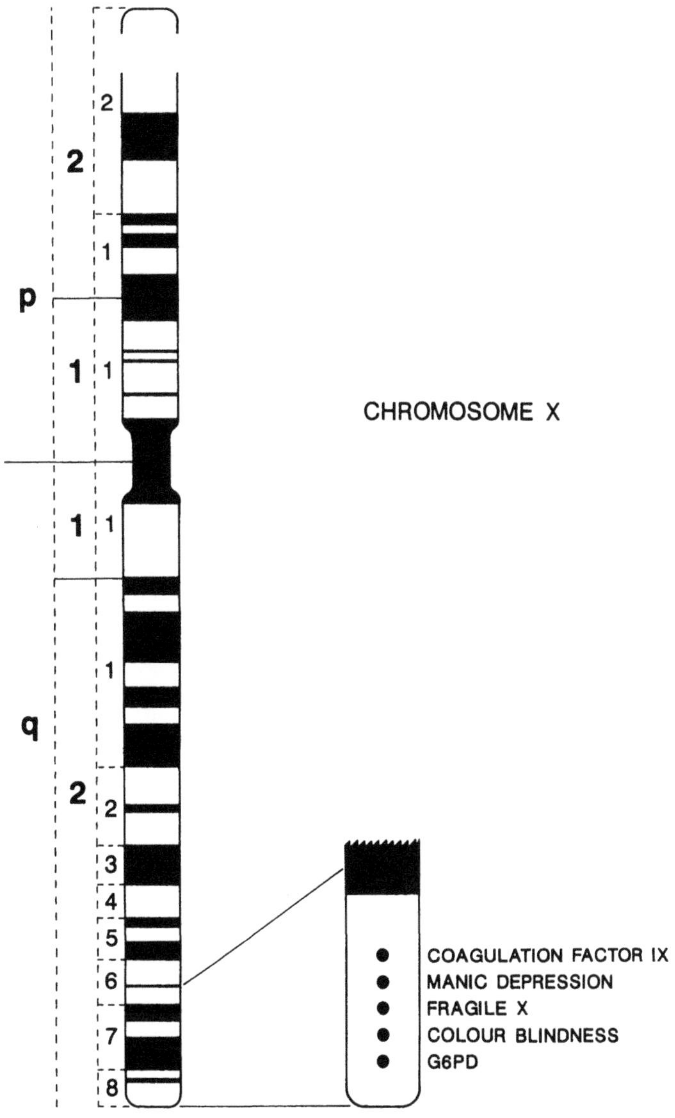

Fig. 2. Map of chromosome X

manic-depressive illness. In the case of schizophrenia, the application of linkage studies using molecular biology and DNA technology also raises important methodological problems because of the probable heterogeneity of the disease. Most twin and family studies, as well as adoption studies, have indicated that schizophrenia seems to have a polygenic mode of transmission, but the involvement of a major gene locus with variable penetrance cannot be excluded. Indeed, there has been a recent report mapping a major gene for schizophrenia in the q11–q13 region of chromosome 5 but unfortunately these findings could not be

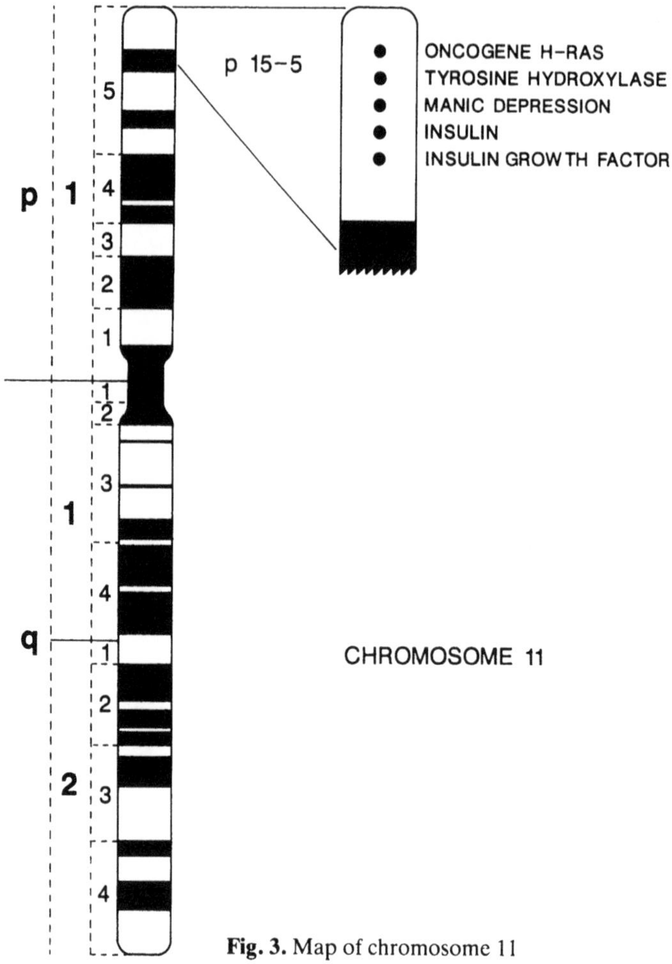

Fig. 3. Map of chromosome 11

confirmed (Kennedy et al. 1988; St. Clair et al. 1989). It is therefore essential to collect more large multiplex kindreds of both schizophrenic and affectively ill probands in different laboratories to confirm previously reported linkages and assess the other chromosomal regions of the human genome with new polymorphic DNA markers. Cytogenetic studies investigating chromosomal anomalies, including translocations or deletion, are also important to consider in future studies, as has been shown by a report showing the presence of a trisomy 5q11-q13 in two schizophrenics in a family of Chinese orgin (Basset et al. 1988). The molecular genetic approach has proven successful in studies on the familial form of Alzheimer's disease. Recent work has drawn attention to clinical and neuropathological similarities between Alzheimer's dementia and the type of dementia observed in late cases of Down's syndrome (Whalley 1982), leading to the localization of a gene on chromosome 21 in the familial form of Alzheimer's disease (St. George-Hyslop et al. 1987), as seen in Fig. 4. However, Alzheimer's disease does not

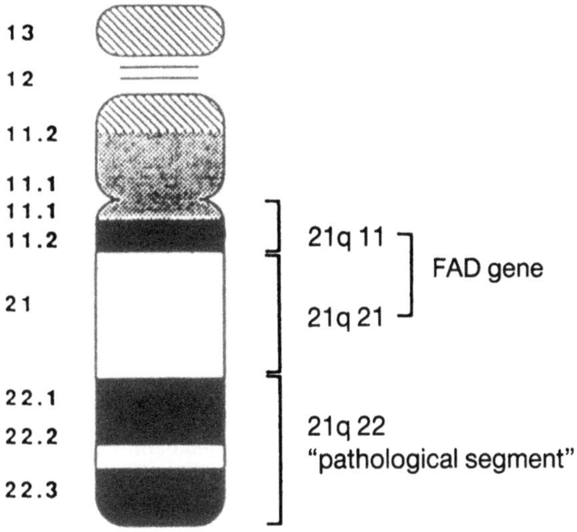

Fig. 4. Chromosome 21: linkage regions for FAD gene (familial Alzheimer's disease) and the pathological segment for Down's syndrome (From Whalley 1987)

segregate with the A4-amyloid gene, also situated on chromsome 21 but not in the vicinity of the Alzheimer gene (Van Broeckhoven et al. 1987).

Other familial forms of Alzheimer's disease do not appear to show linkage on chromosme 21, suggesting that this degenerative illness encompasses different genetic and nongenetic subgroups, as is the case in genetic heterogeneity.

The application of molecular genetics, such as the use of various RFLP and polymerase chain reaction techniques for gene amplification, will provide new powerful tools for data banking of genetic material. The data originating from the behavioral studies in inbred strains of rats could also provide, through chromosomal segregation studies, relevant important information on specific candidate genes and chromosomal markers of neurobiological interest, such as the gene for tyrosine hydroxylase in the 11q region of chromosome 11 (Grima et al. 1985) and the α 3 GABA receptor gene in the Xq 28 region of chromosome X (Schofield et al. 1987), two potential candidate genes in manic-depressive illness to be explored in humans. The discovery of linkage in mental disorders, apart from clarifying the mode of genetic transmission and allowing study of the interaction between genes and other factors in complex behaviors, will also ultimately lead to the isolation, sequencing and cloning of the mutant genes and thus provide some rationale for etiological and preventive therapeutic approaches.

References

Basset AS, McGillivray BC, Jones BD, Tapio Pantzar J (1988) Partial trisomy on chromosome 5 cosegregating with schizophrenia. Lancet I:799–800

Detera-Wadleigh SD, Berretini WH, Goldin LR, Boorman D, Anderson SB, Gershon ES (1987) Close linkage of C-Harvey-ras-1 and the insulin gene to affective disorder is ruled out in three North American pedigrees. Nature 325:806–808

Egeland JA, Gerhard DS, Pauls DL, Sussex JS, Kidd KK, Allen CR, Hostetter AM, Housman DE (1987) Bipolar affective disorders linked to DNA markers on chromosome 11. Nature 325:783–787

Grima B, Lamoureux A, Blanot F. Faucon Biguet N, Mallet J (1985) Complete coding sequence of rat tyrosine hydroxylase mRNA. Proc Natl Acad Sci USA 82:617–621
Hodgkinson S, Sherrington R, Gurling H, Marchbanks R, Reeders S, Mallet J, McInnes M, Petursson H, Brynjolfson (1987) Molecular genetic evidence of heterogeneity in manic-depression. Nature 325:805–806
Kennedy JL, Guiffrat LA, Moises HW, Cavalli-Sforza LL, Pakstis AJ, Kidd JR, Castiglione CM, Sjogren B, Wetterberg L, Kid KK (1988) Evidence against linkage of schizophrenia to markers on chromosome 5 in a northern Swedish pedigree. Nature 336:167–170
Mendlewicz J (1986) X-linked transmission of affective illness: current status and new evidence. In: Shagass C, Josiassen R, Bridger W, Weiss K, Stoff D, Simpson G (eds) Biological psychiatry, vol 7. Elsevier, Amsterdam, pp 46–48
Mendlewicz J (1988) Population and family studies in depression and mania. Br J Psychiatry 153 (Suppl 3):16–25
Mendlewicz J, Rainer J (1977) Adoption study supporting genetic transmission in manic-depressive illness. Nature 268:327–329
Mendlewicz J, Simon P, Charon F, Brocas H, Legros S, Vassart G (1987) A polymorphic DNA marker on X chromosome and manic-depression. Lancet I:1230–1232
Michael G, McKeon P, Humphries P (1988) Linkage analysis of manic depression in an Irish family using H-ras 1 and INS DNA markers. J Med Genet 25:634–637
Schofield PR, Darlison MG, Fujita N, Burt DR, Stefpenson FA, Rodriguez H, Rhee LM, Ramachandran J, Reale V, Glencorse TA, Seeburg PH, Barnard EA (1987) Sequence and functional expression of the $Gaba_A$ receptor shows a ligand-gated receptor super-family. Nature 328:221–227
Sherrington R, Brynjolfsson J, Petursson H, Potter M, Dudleston K, Barraclough B, Wasmuth J, Dobbs M, Gurling H (1988) Localization of a susceptibility locus for schizophrenia on chromosome 5. Nature 336:164–167
St. Clair D, Blackwood D, Muir W, Baillie D, Hubbard A, Wright A, Evans HJ (1989) No linkage of chromosome q11–q13 markers on schizophrenia in Scottish families. Nature 339:305–309
St. George-Hyslop P, Tanzi RE, Polinsky RJ, Haines JL, Nee L, Watkins PC, Myers RH, Feldman RG, Pollen D, Drachman D, Growdon J, Bruni A, Foncin JF, Salmon D, Frommelt P, Amaducci L, Sorbi S, Piacentini S, Stewart GG, Hobbs WJ, Connelly M, Gusella JF (1987) The genetic defect causing familial Alzheimer's disease maps on chromosome 21. Science 235:885–890
Van Broeckhoven C, Genthe AM, Vandenberghe A, Horsthemke B, Backhovens H, Raeymaekers P, Van Hul W, Wehnert A, Gheuens J, Cras P, Bruyland M, Martin JJ, Salbaum M, Multhaup G, Masters CL, Beyreuther K, Gurling HMD, Mullan MJ, Holland A, Barton A, Irving N, Williamson R, Richards SJ, Hardy JA (1987) Failure of familial Alzheimer's disease to segregate with the A4-amyloid gene in several European families. Nature 329:153–156
Whalley LJ (1982) The dementia of Down's syndrome and its relevance to aetiological studies of Alzheimer's disease. Ann NY Acad Sci 396:39–54

Strategies for Understanding the Role of Gene Defects in the Pathogenesis of Mental Disorders

F. E. Bloom

Introduction

Given the results of psychiatric epidemiology, as reviewed in part at this meeting, a search for the biological basis for enhanced susceptibility to psychosis might be fruitfully initiated at the level of the molecular genetic specifications of the brain. One approach to defining the critical elements of such a molecular genetic specification emphasizes the detection and characterization of the proteins underlying the phenotypic properties of brains cells, and the emergent functions attributable to their multicellular ensembles. However, most of the complex features of the human brain's organization are as yet incompletely defined. Furthermore, the essential properties of this brain that enable it to achieve the cognitive, emotional, and other behavioral performance characteristics which signify the symptoms of psychosis are unknown, other than for the increase in cortical mass and the added amount of cortico-cortical interconnectivity that is thereby provided.

Therefore, to begin to develop a research strategy that could potentially illuminate these unknown proteins, functions, and supracellular attributes, we have combined molecular biological, biochemical, and cytological methods to survey the degree to which elements of the mammalian genome are expressed with selectivity in the brain. Our early results (Milner and Sutcliffe 1983; Sutcliffe et al. 1983) suggest that at least half of the genome may be viewed as "brain-specific," and that the number of possible proteins pertinent to brain function are too numerous to examine by routine selection. From that task-defining realization has emerged a still more refined strategy to analyze the molecular basis of functional properties within defined fields of the primate neocortex and during defined stages of brain development. We view the identification of these molecules as a critical step in approaching mechanisms pertinent to characterization of the human brain and its neuropsychiatric dysfunctions. Functional and morphologic properties have been the traditional indices by which neurons and their circuits are classified (Jones and Hendry 1988). While such descriptive schemes document neuronal diversity, they cannot per se account for the variations in properties or the nature of the molecular signals that guide and establish these connections and their functions.

Attempts to clarify the uniquely complex structural organization of the brain were first based on empirically derived cell staining methods supplemented later by more powerful and specific circuit tracing methodologies. During the past decade, these anatomic studies have been powerfully extended by immunocytochemical probes specific for products known or inferred to be produced by neurons or glia. The majority of known neurotransmitter substances and their related metabolic enzymes and receptors are shared between the nervous, endocrine, and immune systems. Although such messenger molecule markers can offer extremely pertinent insights into genetically transmitted diseases of the brain (see Martin 1987), the study of transmitters alone cannot provide a comprehensive approach to the determination of the molecular basis of cellular specificity in the brain because of the high proportion of neurons whose transmitters have not yet been identified.

Attempts to define the specific biochemical properties of the nervous system have generally begun with comparative analysis of its chemical differences with cells of other organ systems, especially with regard to the unique lipids of the brain (Lees and Brostoff 1984) and the transmitter γ-amminobutyrate (see Roberts and Kuriyama 1968). A direct biochemical approach has also been highly successful in identifiying specific molecules based on existing assays of predicted action, such as the hypophysiotrophic hormones (see Guillemin 1978), or based on certain predictable chemical features of transmitter peptides, such as C-terminal amidation (see Tatemoto and Mutt 1980). However, by their specialized nature, it is difficult to infer from these successful applications of an assay-based identification scheme whether or not the specific molecules that were identified represented a large or small proportion of the available physiological regulatory systems of the brain. Although the lists of brain-specific, glia-specific, or neuron-specific molecules that have been detected are growing (see Sutcliffe 1988), one recognizes that we are still in the primitive stages of such list-building, let alone its functional implications.

Molecular Biological Studies on the Rat Brain

We have, therefore, sought a more direct route to the molecular basis by which such neural properties are generated and maintained. Such an alternative approach has only recently become accessible through the powerful methods of recombinant DNA technology. As noted by Sutcliffe (1988), the past 5 years have witnessed an advantageous coupling of the methods of molecular biology to neuroscience. This combination has provided a general solution to the initially overwhelming complexity of the brain by making available rapid and precise means to reduce the enormous numbers of molecules to the many or few that may meet an operational definition of what a specific investigative protocol may wish to define as "interesting". By providing power, speed, precision, and the ability to define the target molecules of interest, mammalian neuroscientists can, in principle, create their preferred model systems for molecular discovery without relinquishing their desire to obtain data on the mammalian brain itself.

Using these methods, the original efforts of our group were directed towards the general issues of whether the special properties of the brain were based upon different proportions of the same proteins and other gene products found in other organs, or whether the special functional properties of the brain derived from genes and gene products that might be regarded as specific for brain function

(Milner and Sutcliffe 1983; see Milner et al. 1987). These brain mRNA complexity studies extended earlier observations (see Kaplan and Finch 1982; Chaudhari and Hahn 1983) that the mammalian brain expresses a large number of distinct mRNAs, expressed exclusively or at least predominantly in the brain as a whole, and in most regions, increasing in abundance in the brains of those species whose brains develop postnatally (see Milner et al. 1987 for more extensive references).

The majority of the clones derived from mRNAs expressed in the adult rat brain, as reported by Milner and Sutcliffe (1983), could be reduced to a few distinct categories, based upon the degree to which these mRNAs were also detectable in the adult liver or kidney. Those defined as class I mRNAs, accounting for approximately 20% of the total, were detectable in approximately identical abundances in brain, liver, and kidney. This category of mRNA may be conceived of as encoding "housekeeping proteins," inferred to be expressed in all cell at approximately the same level. One such example, the cyclosporin-binding protein, "cyclophilin" (Danielson et al. 1988), was detected using this strategy, and has served as a useful internal normalization index of mRNA preparations from a variety of organs and brain regions. A second large class of brain-derived mRNAs reported by Milner and Sutcliffe (1983), or class II, also represented about 20% of the total in brain, and were also present in the liver or kidney, but at abundance estimates that differed significantly across these organs. This class is inferred to represent those mRNAs that encode proteins needed in more than one cell type, but at different concentrations, depenting upon the degree of specialization of the cell and the protein. An example of such mRNAs are those that encode the structural proteins of the tubulin family (also see Miller et al. 1987b).

The third class of brain-derived mRNAs defined by Milner and Sutcliffe (1983), class III, were those detected in brain, but not liver or kidney. Thus, operationally, these mRNAs and their protein products can be regarded as brain-specific. Comparing the three categories of brain-derived mRNAs, Northern blot analyses revealed that those of class III were no longer, by almost twofold, than those of class I, and those class III mRNAs of lesser abundance tended to be the longest of this class. Given that the rarest detectable class III mRNAs averaged about 5000 nucleotides in length, and made up the bulk of those derived from the brain numerically, Milner and Sutcliffe (1983) have estimated that the brain must express at least 30000 genes, of which at least 30% must be regarded as enriched in or selective for the brain.

Using these methods, the specific, but unknown, properties of neurons, both generally and individually, can be approached directly in terms of the gene products expressed in brain, but not in other large, minimally innervated organs (see Sutcliffe et al. 1983, 1984). With this basic organ differential approach, we sought to develop a more general approach to analysis of the molecular basis of brain specificity. We isolated cDNA clones of several mRNAs that are enriched in brain by more than 100 times the limits of detectability for liver and kidney, and determined their nucleotide sequences, thereby obtaining the amino acid sequence of the corresponding proteins by deduction from the genetic code.

The presumptive gene products were then detected using polyclonal antisera raised against selected synthetic fragments of the deduced amino acid sequences (Sutcliffe et al. 1983). In addition to revealing immunocytochemically – defined shared properties of otherwise unrelated neurons in widely separated portions of the rat neuraxis, antisera to the peptide products of these brain-specific mRNAs have also provided useful markers of brain differentiation (Lenoir et al. 1986; Miller et al. 1987a, b) and permit ready comparison across species. A more extensive description of one specific clone analyzed in this fashion may reveal the powers of this strategy and, in particular, how one may initiate an extended analysis of a brain-specific gene product, with no functional preconceptions, when randomly applied to brain-specifice gene analysis.

IB236MAG: An Immunoglobulin-like Brain-specific Cell Adhesion Molecule Expressed in both Neurons and Glia

The rat brain-specific protein 1B236 was originally defined by characterization of randomly selected cDNA clones of mRNAs expressed in adult rat brain, but not detectable in liver or kidney (Milner and Sutcliffe 1983; Sutcliffe et al. 1983). Nucleotide sequence analysis of pIB236 provided the 3′ partial sequence of the mRNA revealing the 3′ end of an open reading frame from which a 318 amino acid putative translation product was deduced. Antisera to each of three synthetic peptides corresponding to nonoverlapping regions of the C-terminus of the IB236 sequences detected at 100 kd rat brain protein containing up to 30 N-linked carbohydrates sites (see also Malfroy et al. 1985). Proteolytic fragments derived from the C-terminus, corresponding to three of the synthetic peptides predicted as possible cleavage products, were also detectable (Malfroy et al. 1985). Both IB236 mRNA and its protein are expressed early in rat brain development, beginning on postnatal day 3 (see Lenoir et al. 1985). Immunocytochemical analysis (Bloom et al. 1985) and in situ hybridization analysis (Higgins et al. 1986, 1989; Lai et al. 1988) showed two phases of developmental expression: during days 3–20, IB236 is expressed predominantly in oligodendrocytes within myelinating tracts throughout the CNS. However, after day 20, IB236 mRNA and protein are detected predominantly in subsets of neurons within gray matter of the olfactory, limbic, motor, and somatosensory systems (Bloom et al. 1986; Higgins et al. 1986, 1989; Lai et al. 1988).

Further analysis revealed that there is only one IB236 gene, but at least two major forms of mRNA that can be derived from it by differential splicing (Lai et al. 1987a). The alternative form also encodes two slightly different forms of the protein product, varying at their C-termini. From the complete primary structure of the two major RNAs forms, we deduced that both protein products have a single transmembrane region, separating a large, highly glycosylated amino terminal region from two alternative carboxyl terminal tails. The shared amino terminal region consists of five, roughly equal sized domains, each encoded by a separate exon, that are closely related in sequence to each other. These domains of internal similarity also reveal further homologies by computer search of previously known protein structures. In particular, IB236 was found to show significant structural similarity to members of the immunoglobulin superfamily (Williams 1987), including the neural cell adhesion molecule, N-CAM (Cunningham et al. 1987) and the platelet-derived growth factor (Yarden et al. 1986; also see Lai et al. 1987b). In addition, through cross-reactivity of in vitro expressed segments of the 1B236 mRNAs, the 1B236 protein is indistinguishable from the so-called myelin associated glycoprotein (MAG), a chemically defined, nervous system-specific glycoprotein expressed by oligodendrocytes during the process of myelination (Quarles 1984) and purported to be functionally related to the interaction between the myelin-producing cells and the axons they myelinate (Martini and Schachner 1986). From the work to date on 1B236/MAG, one recognizes that many brain-specific proteins exist for which no previously conceived functions could have predicted the sorts of bioassays that have classically led to molecular discovery. Given that 1B236 was selected for analysis virtually at random, the likelihood of encountering interesting molecules even when they are studied at random might seem to be reasonably high. From the same series of brain mRNA detection experiments (Sutcliffe et al. 1983) have emerged additional mRNAs that remain under active examination. Among those mRNAs which have continued to maintain our attention are the following representative examples:

p1B1075

p1B1075 is represented by a major and minor form of mRNA, both approximately 2000 nucleotides in length, with an approximate abundance of 0.05%, and encodes an open reading frame that represents a novel protein sequence of approximately 533 amino acids, a high proportion of which are basic and acidic amino acids. Although its regional representation by Northern blot analysis was unremarkable, mapping studies of single-stranded riboprobes labeled with ^{35}S nucleotides for in situ hybridization showed that large neurons of the cortical and subcortical areas were intensely labeled.

pCD42

pCD42 represents a brain-enriched mRNA of approximately 2300 nucleotides in length, that contains an open reading frame for a highly acidic protein of 675 amino acids. Although not detectable in liver or kidney, this mRNA was highly enriched in anterior pituitary and adrenal medulla and on computer search of the sequences was found to have a high degree of similarity to proteins of the secretogranin family (see Forss-Peter et al. 1988). Indeed, when this mRNA was mapped by in situ hybridization, intense labelling was observed over the adrenal medullary chromaffin cells, isolated cells of the anterior pituitary, as well as over distinct clusters of large neurons in several brain structures.

pRC3

pRC3, discovered from a subsequent cDNA library prepared from rat brain poly-A^+ mRNAs, also encodes sequences represented by two mRNAs, one of 1000 nucleotides length and the other of approximately 1500 nucleotides, both of modest abundance. An intriguing feature of this mRNA set is that it is more strongly represented in rodent cortical regions with respect to medullary or pontine structures, and that its open reading frame encodes a novel protein of only 78 amino acids.

Several other mRNAs obtained from these studies of adult rat brain have also been studied and there are literally thousands more to be studied in detail. Thus, it became clear to my colleagues and me that additional strategies were required to focus our attack.

Molecular Biological Analysis of the Primate Neocortex

There is no lack of strategies by which one might begin to analyze the pool of brain-specific mRNAs for those that encode protein products that would assist in the orderly dissection of the cells and cell systems in the brain. For example, Greengard et al. have developed the strategy of detecting proteins that serve as substrates of phosphorylation or dephosphorylation reactions, and have used this approach to characterize several previously undisclosed proteins within definable chemical phenotypes (Walaas et al. 1983a, b). We opted for a strategy more reliant on brain cellular structure, since the past decade's research on neuronal geometry has made clear than even chemically similar neuronal phenotypes can express wide degrees of structural variation, presumed to reflect some uncertain aspect of innervation density (Purves and Lichtmann 1985).

Therefore, we have evolved a strategy from the premise that subsets of neurons defined by their grouping of shared or unique functional features could help define the molecular markers of these functions. By trying to identify the molecular systems underlying the characteristic structural and functional properties of the neurons of the primate cerebral cortex, we sought a more restrictive, but still functionally open-ended approach to identifying cell-specific functional molecules. Certainly, the neocortex is a critical region for understanding the sorts of dysfunctions unique to the human brain, such as the psychoses on which this conference focuses attention. Furthermore, several obvious features of the neocortex were directly relevant for our focused objectives. From our operationally oriented perspective, we viewed the cerebral cortex as a brain region in which vastly differing functional capacities are expressed by neurons arranged in macroscopically homogeneous arrays, that differ only modestly from one region of cortex to another, but in which there are important variations in function, in cytoarchitectonics, and in connectivity properties within functionally definable regions. The added complexity of the primate cerebral cortex, defining even greater regional and subregional specializiations, each having its own more highly refined cytoarchitectonic basis, suggested that this cortex was a highly suitable system in which to exploit molecular biologic approaches to neural cell specificity, as well as being of obvious importance for understanding overall brain function, and cognitive dysfunction.

To apply these properties of primate neocortex to our molecular biological analysis, we have first begun to capture the mRNA species expressed in three arbitrarily selected index regions of the primate neocortex: the visual cortex, the motor cortex, and the prefrontal cortex. These regions are both anatomically distinct and functionally definable; their characteristic laminar specializations reflect differences in neuronal populations, their cell packing, cell connectivity, and other definable properties. Moreover, the individual cellular differences between these regions must a priori arise from differences in their protein constituents (i.e., differences in structural, membrane, and surface proteins) that provide the different functional and structural properties of the cells in these regions. In turn, these differences in proteins must reflect differences among the incidences or proportions of mRNAs. These types of structural, metabolic, and functional properties are the classes of molecular properties that we wish to identify and characterize, and whose translation into specific forms and regulatory mechanisms we hope eventually to understand. Furthermore, with reference to the human neuropsychiatric diseases, such protein markers may be directly useful to probe the pathology of the human brain as novel immunoreagents of neuropathology and also as possible genetic markers in linkage studies of inheritable disorders or traits (see Martin 1987). We anticipated that the extraordinarily well-defined structural and functional subregions of the primate neocortex could facilitate the search for neuron-specific markers that reflect potentially unique properties of individual neurons and the constellation of phenotypes of related neurons.

Primate Cortex-"Specific" mRNAs: Initial Results

Using conventional methods, poly-A^+ mRNA was isolated from young adult male cynomolgus monkeys (see Travis et al. 1987). The initial primate brain cDNA library generated from this RNA yielded more than one million clones, each with an insert frequency of approximately 90% and an insert size ranging from several hundred to at least 6000 mRNAs. Given this imposing number of primate cortex-derived mRNAs, a two-step strategy was devised for selecting those of functional importance for neocortex as compared with cerebellum: first, employing subtractive hybridization methods (cortex-derived ^{32}P-labeled single-stranded cDNAs were hybridized to a large excess of unlabeled cerebellar-derived mRNA from the same specimens) and second, employing differential colony hybridization, with cDNA prepared from either cortex or cerebellum to define those from the first stage studies that were expressed selectively in neocortex (see Travis et al. 1987). One typical run, with approximately 25 000 cDNA clones derived from mRNAs of the adult primate neocortex, yielded first approximately 1200 that were apparently enriched in neocortex over cerebellum, and reduced to less than 50 cDNAs when these "cortex-enriched" clones were further defined with greater sensitivity after being hybridized with probes of cDNAs derived from cerebellum or liver. The resultant set of tentative cortex-specific mRNAs were then screened for intracortical regional abundance variation by performing Northern blots with these clones on mRNAs derived from either visual, motor, or dorsal prefrontal cortex.

Of the first several mRNAs of this last stage results studied in this protocol, five were found by these criteria to be selective for cortex and not detected in cerebellum, one detected mRNAs of different sizes in neocortex and cerebellum, and three others were found in mRNAs of several other brain regions, but relatively reduced in cerebellum. One of those initially regarded as present in cortex and not in cerebellum (termed 1B4 in our protocols) was in fact also found in cerebellum following direct Northern blot analysis with cerebellum-derived cDNA, and at slightly greater overall abundance in motor or dorsal prefrontal cortex as compared with visual cortex, and was later found to be markedly reduced in basal ganglia (see Travis et al. 1987).

Of the initial, independently detected "cortex-specific" clones (compared cerebellum or liver), all five were later found to hybridize to target mRNAs of approximately the same size and with an abundance of approximately 0.05%, and all five showed cross-hybridization on Southern blot analysis, indicating that they represented the same brain-specific, cortex-specific gene, termed 1H8A in our protocols (see Travis et al. 1987). To define in greater spatial precision the cellular sites in which these cortex-enriched mRNAs were expressed, we applied in situ hybridization using ^{35}S plasmid-derived DNA. Clone 1H8A detected mRNAs in subpopulations of cells, in laminae II–VI, in all cortical regions examined, with slightly higher densities in prefrontal regions over temporal regions. Clone 1B4, although not meeting our desire for cortical exclusivity, did on in situ hybridization analysis show far greater selective spatial distribution across cortical regions and laminae. Labelling of cells was most dense in laminae V and VI of the primary visual region (area 17) of the occipital lobe, and in the inferior temporal gyrus of the temporal lobe, as well as in layered neurons of the underlying lateral geniculate nucleus (see Travis et al. 1987).

More recently, using still further refinements of this two-step subtractive differential hybridization approach (Travis and Sutcliffe 1988), the overall sensitivity of the method has been further increased to extend the threshold for detection down to at least 0.001% of the total mRNA. Following this methodological improvement, it has again been possible to identify cortex-derived mRNAs not apparently expressed in cerebellum. An initial breakdown of 100 clones meeting this operational, differential region detection criterion (Travis and Sutcliffe, personal communication) indicates that approximately 93 isolates were again representing the mRNA of 1H8A (with an overall abundance of 0.05% or more). Of the other seven primate cortex-derived isolates, whose abundance approaches the current theoretical threshold of 0.001%, six have undergone initial nucleotide sequence analysis, revealing that two represented the neuropeptides somatostatin and cholecystokinin, known to be absent from cerebellum, as well as four other unique sequences of approximately the same abundance. The latter show some regional variations within cortex on Northern blot analyses, but none so far analyzed can be regarded as unique to any primate neocortical region. These cDNAs remain under active investigation as to their cellular distributions. In all cases, detailed regional as well as cellular mapping, both with in situ hybridization as well as by immunocytochemistry with antisera raised against the gene product, will be necessary to draw any definitive conclusions regarding breadth or selectivity of their distribution.

Based upon the data presently in hand, a very conservative interpretation of the results would take the view that, thus far, no "cell-type" specific mRNAs have been detected by our approaches. If this conclusion is supported by further observations, it would suggest that the obvious and dramatic differences in neuronal cytology, circuitry, and signaling systems are based upon recombinations in varying proportions, and with varying representations of members of the rare to very rare classes of brain mRNAs, with many proteins, even those defined as neuron-specific being represented more frequently and most broadly. Given this array of common, less common, and rare mRNAs, some of which have begun to be defined by our methods as region-specific, one might still speculate that such region-specific gene products could provide important determinants on the neurons within that region.

Conclusions

At this stage in the evolution of the neurosciences, molecular and cellular research in combination provide a progressive, interactive series of research strategies potentially capable of defining specific neuronal phenotypic markers, and the developmental patterns by which they are expressed uniquely, as well as the possible principles by which they may be shared. The strategies we have undertaken to develop have certain operational advantages in conceptualization of disorders, such as the psychoses, in which the nature of the underlying factors enhancing susceptibility to express the signs and the symptoms of the disorder must be based on abnormalities within the CNS. Furthermore, it is our contention that identification of brain-specific gene products without bioassay filters for the discovery process can in fact reveal new cellular functions and novel molecularly based concepts of brain organization. Among the classes of known CNS proteins that have been established as the underlying defects in genetically linked behavioral abnormalities are the hypocerebellar mouse mutant *jimpy,* whose problems arise from defective myelination during development (see references in Nave et al. 1987a, b).

Given the prominence of myelin-derived proteins in the CNS, it was not unexpected that our initial studies of the most enriched of the brain-specific mRNAs should in fact lead to the proteins of the myelin. In fact, among our earliest brain-specific clones was one (p1B208; Sutcliffe et al. 1983) which was later established to be myelin proteolipid (see Milner et al. 1987). When we were able to isolate one of the two alternatively spliced forms of the myelin proteolipid mRNA from a mouse cDNA library, it was then possible to obtain a rather detailed view of the normal gene and to compare the normal with its counterpart, established by us to be approximately a 74 nucleotide deletion (see Nave et al. 1987a, b) isolated from a cDNA library from the *jimpy* mutation. Analysis of the *jimpy* proteolipid gene established that the missing segment is equivalent to a single exon, and that at the 3′ end of the adjacent intron, a single nucleotide base alteration (from adenine to guanine) led to the formation of a splice acceptor site, and to the abnormal processing of the mRNA, leading in turn to defective myelin formation as a result of a missing protein.

Another example from our studies is one that may perhaps be more closely related to the type of very subtle changes that could be viewed as pertinent to models of psychosis gene transmission. In studies of gene expression in the postnatally developing rat hypothalamus, using the mRNA for the oxytocin gene as a probe, we have observed that there is a marked gender-based and hormone-sensitive regulation of this neuropeptide, such that the male brains are far richer and have many more neurons expressing the oxytocin mRNA, while in the female, puberty regulates the amount of oxytocin expression in a restricted number of neurons (Miller et al. 1988, 1989). Since at least one of the forms of chronic schizophrenia has been classically linked to brain changes beginning at or near puberty, it is reasonable to consider that far greater definition of these effects of gonadal maturation on the brain must be pursued.

A comprehensive strategy to elucidate the molecular basis of neuronal specificity thus constitutes an important long-term goal of our research program. As a part of the broadly based strategies currently evolving to link genetic markers with complex human disorders, we take the view that any of the thousands of still-to-be-discovered brain-specific genes could provide a genomic mapping marker of direct CNS pertinence, and that this same application could be made with perhaps more emphasis for those that can be further characterized as region-specific. Given the very large number of gene defects that can result in "mental retardation" states (see Gurling 1986), it may be presumed that normal cognitive ability must depend on a very large array of gene products. Given that the incidence of the major psychoses can be linked only partially to inheritable factors, we intend to persist in our general strategy. While we are sanguine that cell-specific markers may not be definable yet by these methods, should they exist, it remains likely that knowledge of brain-specific and region-specific mRNAs will nevertheless offer important insight into the organizational and functional complexity of the brain.

Acknowledgments. This work was supported by NIH Grants NS 22347 and NS 20728. This paper is BCR 5960.

References

Bloom FE; Battenberg ELF, Milner RJ, Sutcliffe JG (1985) Immunocytochemical mapping of 1B236, brain specific neuronal polypeptide deduced from the sequence of a cloned mRNA. J Neurosci 5:1781–1802

Bloom FE, Battenberg E, Milner RJ and Sutcliffe JG (1986) Molecular biology and histochemical mapping of the nervous system. In: Neurohistochemistry: Modern Methods and Applications, Alan R. Liss, Inc., pp 3–19

Chaudhari N, Hahn WE (1983) Genetic expression in the developing brain. Science 220:924–928

Cunningham BA, Hemperly JJ, Murray BA, Prediger E, Brackenbury R, Edelman GM (1987) Neural cell adhesion molecule: structure, immunoglobulin-like domains, cell surface modulation, and alternative RNA splicing. Science 236:799–806

Danielson PE, Forss-Petter S, Brown MA, Calavetta L, Douglass J, Milner RJ, Sutcliffe JG (1988) p1B15: a cDNA clone of the rat mRNA encoding cyclophilin. DNA 7:261–267

Forss-Petter S, Travis G, Milner RJ, Bloom FE, Sutcliffe JG (1989) Gene expressions in the mammalian brain. In: Vartanian M (ed) Neuronal receptors, endogenous ligands and biotechnical approaches (in press)

Guillemin R (1978) Peptides in the brain: the new endocrinology of the neuron. Science 202:390–398

Gurling H (1986) Candidate genes and favoured loci: Strategies for molecular genetic research into schizophrenia, manic depression, autism, alcoholism, and Alzheimer's Disease. Psychiatr Dev 4:289–309

Higgins GA, Schmale H, Bloom FE, Wilson MC, Milner RJ (1986) Developmental shift in the cellular expression of the brain-specific gene 1B236: Localization to oligodendrocytes revealed by in situ hybridization. Soc Neurosci Abstr 12:213

Higgins GA, Schmale H, Bloom FE, Wilson MC, Milner RJ (1989) Cellular localization of 1B236/myelin-associated glycoprotein (1B236/MAG) mRNA during rat brain development. Proc Natl Acad Sci USA 86:2074–2078

Jones EG, Hendry SHC (1988) Expression of neuronal diversity in the central nervous system. In: Jones EG (ed) Molecular biology of the human brain. UCLA Symp Mol Cell Biol 72:3–12

Kaplan BB, Finch CE (1982) The sequence complexity of brain ribonucleic acids. In: Brown IR (ed) Molecular approaches to neurobiology Academic, New York, pp 71–98

Lai C, Brow MA, Nave KA, Noronha AB, Quarles R, Bloom FE, Milner RJ, Sutcliffe JG (1987a) Two putative cell adhesion molecules for postnatal neuronal development produced by alternative splicing of the 1B236/myelin-associated glycoprotein (MAG) gene. Proc Natl Acad Sci USA 84:4337–4341

Lai C, Watson J, Bloom FE, Sutcliffe JG, Milner RJ (1987b) The neural protein 1B236/MAG defines a subpopulation of the immunoglobulin superfamily. Imm Rev 100:129–151

Lai C, Battenberg ELF, Milner RT, Bloom FE (1988) 1B236/MAG expression in neurons. Soc Neurosci Abstr 14:1267

Lees MB, Brostoff SW (1984) Proteins of myelin. In: Morell P (ed) Myelin. Plenum, New York, pp 197–224

Lenoir D, Battenberg E, Kiel M, Bloom FE, Milner RJ (1986) The brain-specific gene 12B36 is expressed postnatally in the developing rat brain. J Neurosci 6:522–530

Malfroy B, Bakhit C, Bloom FE, Sutcliffe JG, Milner RJ (1985) Brain-specific polypeptide 1B236 exists in multiple molecular forms. Proc Natl Acad Sci USA 82:2009–2013

Martin JB (1987) Molecular genetics: applications to the clinical neurosciences. Science 238:765–772

Martini R, Schachner A (1986) Immunoelectron microscopic localization of neural cell adhesion molecules (L1, N-CAM, and MAG) and their shared carbohydrate epitope and myelin basic protein in developing sciatic nerve. J Cell Biol 103:2439–2448

Miller FD, Naus CCG, Higgins GA, Bloom FE, Milner RJ (1987a) Developmentally regulated rat brain mRNAs: molecular and anatomical characterization. J Neurosci 7:2433–2444

Miller FD, Naus CCG, Higgins GA, Bloom FE, Milner RJ (1987b) Isotypes of alpha-tubulin are differentially regulated during neuronal maturation. J Cell Biol 105:3065–3073

Miller FD, Milner RJ, Bloom FE (1988) Neuronal oxytocin mRNA regulation by gonadal steroids in developing adult rats. Soc Neurosci Abstr 14:

Miller FD, Ozimek G, Milner RJ, Bloom FE (1989) Regulation of neuronal oxytocin mRNA by ovarian steroids in the mature and developing hypothalamus. Proc Natl Acad Sci USA 86:2468–2472

Milner RJ, Sutcliffe JG (1983) Gene expression in rat brain. Nucleic Acids Res 11:5497–5520

Milner RJ, Bloom FE, Sutcliffe JG (1987) Brain specific genes: strategies and issues. Curr Top Dev Biol 21:117–150

Nave KA, Lai C, Bloom FE, Milner RJ (1987a) Splice site selection in the proteolipid protein (PLP) gene transcript and primary structure of the DM-20 protein of central nervous system myelin. Proc Natl Acad Sci USA 84:5665–5669

Nave KA, Lai C, Bloom FE, Milner RJ (1987b) A single nucleotide difference in the gene for myelin proteolipid protein defines the *jimpy* mutation in mouse. J Neurochem 49:1873–1877

Purves D, Lichtman J (1985) Geometrical differences among homologous neurons in mammals. Science 228:298–305

Quarles RH (1984) Myelin-associated glycoprotein in development and disease. Dev Neurosci 6:285–303

Roberts E, Kuriyama K (1968) Biochemical-physiological correlations in studies of the gamma-aminobutyric acid system. Brain Res 8:1–37

Sutcliffe JG (1988) mRNA in the brain mammalian central nervous system. Annu Rev Neurosci 11:157–198

Sutcliffe JG, Milner RJ, Shinnick TM, Bloom FE (1983) Identifiying the protein products of brain-specific genes with antibodies to chemically synthesized peptides. Cell 33:671–682

Sutcliffe JG, Milner RJ, Gottesfeld JM, Reynolds W (1984) Control of neuronal gene expression. Science 225:1308–1315
Tatemoto K, Mutt V (1980) Isolation of two novel candidate hormones using an ethical method for finding naturally occuring polypeptides. Nature 285:417–419
Travis GH (1987) Substractive cDNA cloning and analysis of primate neocortex mRNAs with regionally-heterogenous distributions. Neuropharmacology 26:845–854
Travis G, Sutcliffe JG (1988) Phenol emulsion-enhanced DNA-driven subtractive cDNA cloning; isolation of low-abundance monkey cortex-specific mRNAs. Proc Natl Acad Sci USA 85:1696–1700
Travis GH, Naus CCG, Morrison JH, Sutcliffe JG (1986) Complementary DNA cloning of heterogeneously distributed monkey cortex RNAs. Soc Neurosci Abstr 12:1457
Walaas SI, Nairn AC, Greengard P (1983a) Regional distribution of calcium- and cyclic adenosine 3′:5′-monophosphate-regulated protein phosphorylation systems in mammalian brain. I. Particulate systems. J Neurosci 3:291–301
Walaas SI, Nairn AC, Greengard P (1983b) Regional distribution of calcium- and cyclic adenosine 3′:5′-monophosphate-regulated protein phosphorylation systems in mammalian brain. II. Soluble systems. J Neurosci 3:302–313
Williams AF, Barclay AN, Clark MJ, Gagnon J (1985) Cell surface glycoproteins and the origin of immunity. In: Anderson LC, Gahmberg CG, Ekblom P (eds) Gene expression during normal and malignant differentation. Academic Press, London. pp 125–138
Williams AF (1987) A year in the life of the immunoglubulin super-family. Immunol Today 8:298–303
Yarden Y, Escobedo JA, Kuang WJ, Yang-Feng TL, Daniel TO, Tremble PM, Chen EY, Ando ME, Harkins R, Frencke U, Fried VA, Ullrich A, Williams LT (1986) Structure of the receptor for platelet-derived growth factor helps define a family of closely related growth factor receptors. Nature 323:226–232

The Identification of Genes which Cause or Predispose to Mental Illness

R. Williamson and *A. M. Goate*

Summary

The first step in demonstrating a genetic component to a disease is usually to show linkage between polymorphic DNA markers and the disease in multiply affected families. Linkage analysis in such families permits the localisation of the genetic defect to a subchromosomal region of 2–10 cm, depending on the number and quality of the pedigrees. Several techniques have been developed to bridge the gap between the resolution of genetic mapping and the identification of the genetic defect which either causes, or predisposes to, a particular mental illness. These include the use of cell lines containing single human chromosomes or chromosome fragments, the isolation of yeast artificial chromosome (YAC) clones or contiguous cosmids covering the region between flanking markers, long-range physical mapping with pulsed-field gel electrophoresis and the isolation of coding genes through library cross-screening or the identification of HTF islands.

The techniques of "reverse genetics" have now been used successfully to identify the genes which, when mutated, cause two X-linked disorders; Duchenne muscular dystrophy and chronic granulomatous disease (Monaco et al. 1986; Royer-Pokora et al. 1986) and the autosomal recessive disorder cystic fibrosis (Rommens et al. 1989). Similar techniques have also been used to identify the chromosomal location to within several hundred kilobases, of the gene causing the autosomal dominant disorder, Huntington's disease (Wasmuth et al. 1988). It is anticipated that the mutant allele causing this disease will probably be identified within the next few years.

The successful application of molecular genetics to the study of these fully penetrant single-gene disorders has encouraged the study of diseases with more complex genetics, such as heart disease, cancer and many mental illnesses.

Several of the most common mental illnesses, including schizophrenia, bipolar affective disorder and Alzheimer's disease (AD), have been shown to have a genetic component to their susceptibility (Murray et al. 1986; Bertelson 1979; Heyman et al. 1983). Multiply affected families in which development of the disease appears to show mendelian inheritance have been described for several mental illnesses, including schizophrenia (Sherrington et al. 1988; Kennedy et al. 1988), bipolar affective disorder (Egeland and Hostetter 1983), Huntington's disease (Wexler et al. 1984) and AD (Nee et al. 1983). These can be used for genetic linkage studies to identify chromosomal localisation of the genetic defect.

Many highly polymorphic DNA markers have now been identified throughout the human genome, so that, given sufficient numbers of affected pedigrees, it is possible to screen the entire genome systematically to look for linkage (Lander and Botstein 1986). However, this process can be considerably shortened if the literature is first surveyed for descriptions of chromosomal translocations, duplications or deletions which appear to have resulted in the development of disease, since these provide candidate chromosomes to test. For example, the clue which led to the detection of linkage between AD and chromosome 21 was the presence of AD neuropathology in virtually all individuals with Down's syndrome over the age of 30 (Oliver and Holland 1986), and the finding of linkage in schizophrenia followed the report of a family in which a schizophrenic illness was segregating with an unbalanced translocation of chromosome 5 (Bassett et al. 1988).

Linkage has now been reported to chromosome 4 for Huntington's disease (Gusella et al. 1983), chromosomes 11 and X for manic depression (Egeland et al. 1987; Mendlewicz et al. 1980), chromosome 21 for AD (St. George-Hyslop et al. 1987; Goate et al. 1989) and chromosome 5 for schizophrenia (Sherrington et al. 1988). However, all but the Huntington's disease linkage are the subject of dispute since other groups have failed to detect linkage at the same loci in different families (Schellenberg et al. 1988; Pericak-Vance et al. 1988; Kennedy et al. 1988; St. Clair et al. 1989; Hodgkinson et al. 1987; Detera-Wadleigh et al. 1987). The failure to detect linkage in these studies has been interpreted as evidence for nonallelic genetic heterogeneity or aetiologic heterogeneity. However, alternative explantations are that either the original linkage was spurious, or that the failure to find linkage was incorrect due to misdiagnosis, phenocopies of the disease within the pedigree or incomplete penetrance (St. George Hyslop et al. 1988). Indeed, recently more individuals have been genotyped for chromosome 11 probes in the Old Order Amish pedigree with affective disorder. Extension of the pedigree and changes in the clinical status of several individuals has led to a decrease in the lod score and exclusion around the original loci used, suggesting that the original result was spurious (Kelsoe et al. 1989).

Usually, when a linkage is detected, it will first be to a single informative DNA probe. If linkage to this probe is real, then other probes from the same region of the chromosome will also detect linkage in the same group of families. It is very useful to have at least one probe that is highly informative, such as a VNTR or $(AC)_n$ repeat probe (Nakamura et al. 1987; Weber and May 1989), which can act as a pivotal point for all families studied. To reduce the possibility of genetic heterogeneity and therefore increase the likelihood of detecting linkage, many small pedigrees should be used. Large families from isolated populations should be excluded from the analysis until a linkage has been detected. Established methods can then be used to test for linkage, and for genetic heterogeneity if linkage cannot be detected.

Probes from Salt Lake City and Collaborative Research are particularly useful since their relative order has been well established using the CEPH families (Donis-Keller et al. 1987; White et al. 1987). At this stage, multipoint linkage analysis in the families can be used to determine the most likely position of the disease locus within the known marker map. This analysis is more robust to uncertainty of probe-probe distance than to mistakes in probe order (Ott 1986). In this way, flanking probes can be identified which delineate the subchromosomal region of interest. In homogeneous disorders for which three-generation pedigrees can be sampled, it should be possible to obtain flanking probes within two cM of the disease locus, that is, with a probable probe-probe distance of less than 5 Mb. The resolution of this genetic mapping is obviously dependent on several factors, including the frequency of misdiagnosis, penetrance, genetic heterogeneity of the disease and pedigree structure (in diseases of late onset, samples are frequently only available from affected individuals in a single generation, reducing considerably the statistical value of each family for linkage analysis; (St. George-Hyslop et al. 1988). All three of these factors are likely to affect analysis in mental illnesses.

When linkage has been established between a disease and markers on a specific chromosome, a set of techniques applicable to any disease is then used to move "from linkage to gene", and to identify the genetic defect. The approach and problems will in essence be similar to those encountered for cystic fibrosis, Huntington's disease or Duchenne muscular dystrophy.

Atypical families or individuals can be useful at this stage, particularly those who have a chromosomal deletion or translocation in the region and are affected by the mental disorder and other conditions, such as mental retardation. For Duchenne muscular dystrophy, Kunkel et al. (1985) showed elegantly how such cases can provide a useful short cut to gene identification.

Another useful resource is a rodent/human hybrid cell line containing only the human chromosome of interest or a suitable subchromosomal fragment. There are now cell lines which contain most human chromosomes singly in a mouse or Chinese hamster background. These cell lines are excellent starting material for constructing specialised libraries, such as "jumping" and "linking" libraries which are particularly useful in conjunction with pulsed-field gel electrophoresis (Poutska and Lehrach 1986; Barlow and Lehrach 1987). Libraries constructed from these cell lines are the best starting points for the isolation of new polymorphic markers mapping close to the disease locus. However, it should be noted that many hybrid cell lines have only been characterised using chromosome-specific *biochemical* markers (rather than DNA), and therefore may contain other human chromosome fragments which have not been detected by this technique.

Another freely available resource is the chromosome-specific phage and cosmid libraries (from ATTC), which were prepared by the Lawrence Livermore Laboratory from flow-sorted chromosomes and are fairly free of contaminants. If the most tightly linked markers are of small sequence length, and not particularly informative for RFLPs, corresponding cosmids and phages can be isolated from these libraries and screened for highly polymorphic elements such as $(AC)_n$ repeats or HTF islands, the CpG-rich islands found at the 3′ or 5′ prime end of genes (Bird 1986).

Once flanking markers have been identified, it is necessary to construct a map of the region using pulsed-field gel electrophoresis to determine the physical distance between the flanking markers. As new markers are isolated they can be placed quickly on the map to determine whether they lie closer to the disease locus. Since many of the "rare cutter" enzymes used for pulsed-field mapping have recognition sequences containing the CpG dinucleotide, they are sensitive to differences in methylation. This can be useful in mapping since the methylation status of different tissues and cell types will give different fragment sizes. If two probes are likely to be separated by several megabases, then hypomethylated cells such as hybrid cell lines are useful, as restriction fragments will tend to be larger due to the absence of some methylation-sensitive sites. In contrast, if several probes are thought to be very close together, then cells from hypermethylated tissues such as sperm can be used to determine the probe order.

If a pulsed-field map is constructed in both normal and affected individuals, it is possible that a deletion, insertion or other rearrangement may be recognised in affected individuals (Den Dunnen et al. 1987). However, if the map does not meet in the middle (that is, the flanking markers are more than four or five Mb apart), more probes from the region will need to be isolated.

For diseases such as cystic fibrosis, genetic mapping using crossovers involving a family member with the disease has been a very powerful tool, allowing the cystic fibrosis gene to be localised to less then one cM. The crossover families must show linkage on one side and a failure of linkage on the other to be considered correct. Once a proven recombination is "crossed" by a new probe, it limits the disease absolutely and sets a closer boundary with a new flanking marker, provided that the diagnosis of the critical individuals was correct and that the disease was fully penetrant.

However, for many mental illnesses where there is evidence for genetic heterogeneity, genetic mapping using crossover families will be less useful, as it will probably not be possible to generate big enough lod scores in individual families to demonstrate linkage on one side of the crossover and failure of linkage of the other. Consequently, alternative explanations of apparent crossovers will always be genetic heterogeneity, incomplete penetrance and ambiguities in diagnosis leading to a decrease in the resolution of genetic mapping. In most mental illnesses it is likely that the resolution of genetic mapping techniques will be of the order of 10 cM (an order of magnitude less than that for cystic fibrosis). This means that isolation of the mutant alleles in psychiatric diseases will rely much more on the use of physical mapping techniques.

A directed "jump" towards the disease locus from either flanking marker can be made by either cloning a fragment from a pulsed-field gel or by screening a jumping library. Markers mapping close to the cystic fibrosis locus have been isolated by cloning a fragment hybridising to the *met* oncogene from a preparative field inversion gel (Michiels et al. 1987).

There are two kinds of jumping libraries, those which jump from rare cutter site to rare cutter site (Poutska and Lehrach 1986) and those which make jumps of 100–200 kb per step using random partial digest libraries (Collins and Weissman 1984). Rare cutter jumping and linking libraries are particularly useful when combined with pulsed-field mapping since they allow one to jump from one HTF island, and therefore candidate gene, to the next between the flanking markers. In Huntington's disease this approach has been used to move 350 kb in a single jump rather than the 10–20 steps required by identifying overlapping cosmids (Poutska et al. 1987; Richards et al. 1988). A detailed pulsed-field map between two flanking markers will identify the position of HTF islands in the region. However, this strategy will not identify all candidate genes since not all genes have HTF islands (Bird 1986).

In diseases such as cystic fibrosis, where a single ancient mutation event is thought to account for most of the cases in northern Europe, linkage disequilibrium exists between marker probes and the disease (Estivill et al. 1987b). Linkage disequilibrium is indicated if the allele frequency of "disease-associated chromosomes" differs from that of the "normal population." This type of calculation is much more difficult than it sounds, and anyone wishing to attempt disequilibrium analysis would be well advised to take expert advice; in particular, the comparison with a "normal population" which is appropriate rarely corresponds with the collection of lab staff whom one often uses for allele frequency determinations.

The next step is to identify all the possible coding sequences, and therefore candidate genes, between the flanking markers. We assume that most of the mutations which cause, or predispose to, a mental (or physical) illness will occur in coding genes. (This is an act of faith to some extent, but is probably the best way to proceed). All the material between the flanking markers should now be cloned, and mapped using pulsed-field gel electrophoresis to identify coding sequences from the region.

Ordered YAC or cosmid clones between the flanking markers is the most economical first step. For example, if flanking markers are 200 kb apart, then a single YAC clone (100–700 kb) may be isolated, containing both flanking markers and the disease locus (Burke et al. 1987). Alternatively, contiguous cosmids (35–50 kb) covering this area may be isolated (at least seven cosmids with 30% overlap would be required). YAC or cosmid libraries can be constructed from a cell line containing only a small fragment of appropriate human chromosome material, or from fragments cloned directly from a pulsed-field gel. In the case of mental illnesses, YAC clones will probably be more appropriate since the flanking markers are likely to be a much larger distance apart.

There are several ways of identifying coding sequences within a stretch of genomic DNA. HTF islands, identified by pulsed-field mapping, are frequently found at the 3′ and 5′ end of genes (Bird 1986). However, while almost all HTF island identify genes, not all genes have HTF islands. The sizes of exons vary, and many are so small that even sequencing does not give a definitive open reading frame. Cosmid or YAC clones must, therefore, be subcloned and fragments containing unique sequences identified and then screened on zooblots to identify those containing conserved sequences. cDNA libraries can then be screened to isolate homologous clones. In general, unless automated DNA sequencing advances rapidly during the next year or two, it would be uneconomical to sequence genomic DNA in the absence of (at least) an indication that a coding gene is present in the region.

cDNA clones should be tested on Northern blots containing mRNA from different human tissues and different brain regions to determine whether the expression pattern of the candidate clone is consistent with that expected from the gene causing the disease. Obviously, in mental illness, brain regions which show the most severe pathology might be expected to express a gene that is mutated so as to cause a disease, for example the hippocampus and amygdala in AD or the caudate putamen in Huntington's disease. It may be important to test mRNA isolated from tissue at different stages during development, since it has been suggested that diseases such as schizophrenia may result from a subtle neurodevelopmental abnormality. However, the mutated gene might well be expressed elsewhere as well, or more important, might be transcirbed at very low levels, even in the brain.

Once a cDNA has been isolated, it is first necessary to prove that it really does map to the region of the chromosome known to be involved, since spurious cross-hybridisation can sometimes be a problem. Next, it must be sequenced and compared between affected and unaffected individuals for differences in sequence and expression levels. Ultimately, it is essential to show that a gene is involved at the functional level. This may be obvious from the predicted protein sequence (for instance, if there is homology with known neurotransmitters, their receptors or relevant enzymes).

For the successful isolation of alleles causing or predisposing to mental illness, advances in technology leading to the easy identification of coding sequence are needed since the distance between flanking markers, and therefore the number of candidate genes, will be much larger. It is likely that transgenic animal experiments will be necessary to demonstrate that a mutation in a particular gene is sufficient to cause the disease. The results of such experiments may be difficult to interpret for mental illness unless there is a biological marker which is definitive for the disease. If such markers can be identified, it is possible that, in the near future, transfection of YAC or cosmid clones into embryonic stem cells, followed by the formation of transgenic mice, may be a feasible method to detect large fragments of DNA (up to 700 kb) containing the disease locus. This may be particularly useful for dominant disorders where misdiagnosis, incomplete pentrance or genetic heterogeneity make it difficult to use crossovers in affected pedigrees to delineate a small region containing the disease locus.

Acknowledgements. This work was supported by the Medical Research Council and the charity Research into Ageing.

References

Barlow D, Lehrach H (1987) Genetics by gel electrophoresis: the impact of pulsed-field gel electrophoresis on mammalian genetics. Trends Genet 3:167–171

Bassett AS, Jones BD, McGillivray BC, Pantzar JT (1988) Partial trisomy chromosome 5 cosegregating with schizophrenia. Lancet I:799–801

Bertelson (1979) A Danish twin study of manic depressive disorders. In: Schou M, Stromgren E (eds) Origin, prevention and treatment of affective disorders. Academic, London, pp 227–239

Bird AP (1986) CpG-rich islands and the function of DNA methylation. Nature 321:209–213

Burke DT, Carle GF, Olson MV (1987) Cloning of large segments of exogenous DNA into yeast by means of artificial chromosome vectors. Science 236:806–812

Collins FS, Weissman S (1984) Directional cloning of DNA fragments at a large distance from an initial probe: a circularisation method. Proc Natl Acad Sci USA 81:6812–6816

Den Dunnen JT, Bakker E, Klein Breiteler EG, Pearson PL, van Ommen GJB (1987) DMD: direct detection of more than 50% of the mutations by field inversion gel electrophoresis. Nature 329:640–642

Detera-Wadleigh SD, Berrettini WH, Goldin LR, Boorman D, Anderson S, Gershon ES (1987) Close linkage of c-Harvey-ras-1 and the insulin gene to affective disorder is ruled out in three North American pedigrees. Nature 325:806–808

Donis-Keller H, Green P, Helms C, Cartinhour S, Weiffenbach B, Stephens K, Keith TP, Bowden DW, Smith DR, Lander ES, Botstein D, Akots G, Rediker KS, Gravius T, Brown VA, Rising MB, Parker C, Powers JA, Watt DE, Kauffman ER, Bricker A, Phipps P, Muller-

Kahle H, Fulton TR, Ng S, Schumm JW, Braman JC, Knowlton RG, Barker DF, Crooks SM, Lincoln S, Daly M, Abrahamson J (1987): A genetic linkage map of the human genome. Cell 51:319–337

Egeland JA, Hostetter AM (1983) Amish studies. I. Affective disorders among the Amish, 1976–1980. Am J Psychiatry 140:56–61

Egeland JA, Gerhard DS, Pauls DL, Sussex JN, Kidd KK, Allen CR, Hostetter AM, Housman DE (1987) Bipolar affective disorders linked to DNA markers on chromosome 11. Nature 325:783–787

Estivill X, Farrall M, Scambler PJ, Bell GM, Hawley KMF, Lench NJ, Bates GP, Kruyer HC, Frederick PA, Stanier P, Watson EK, Williamson R, Wainwright BJ (1987a) A candidate for the cystic fibrosis locus isolated by selection for methylation-free islands. Nature 326:840–845

Estivill X, Scambler PJ, Wainwright BJ, Hawley K, Frederick P, Schwartz M, Baiget M, Kere J, Williamson R, Farrall M (1987b) Patterns of polymorphism and linkage disequilibrium for cystic fibrosis. Genomics 1:257–263

Gusella JF, Wexler NS, Conneally PM, Naylor SL, Anderson A, Tanzi RE, Watkins PC, Ottina K, Wallace MR, Sakaguchi AY, Young AB, Shoulson I, Bonilla E, Martin JB (1983) A polymorphic DNA marker genetically linked to Huntington's disease. Nature 306:234–238

Goate AM, Haynes AR, Owen MJ, Farrall M, James LA, Lai LY-C, Mullan MJ, Roques P, Rossor NM, Williamson R, Hardy JA (1989) Predisposing locus to Alzheimer's disease on chromosome 21. Lancet I:352–355

Heyman A, Wilkinson WE, Hurwith BJ (1983) Alzheimer's disease: genetic aspects and associated clinical disorders. Ann Neurol 14:507–515

Hodgkinson S, Sherrington R, Gurling H, Marchbanks R, Reeders S, Mallet J, McInnis M, Petursson H, Brynjolfsson J (1987) Molecular genetic evidence for heterogeneity in manic depression. Nature 325:805–806

Kelsoe JR, Ginns EI, Egeland JA, Gerhards DS, Goldstein AM, Bale SJ, Pauls DL, Long RT, Kidd KK, Conte G, Housman DE, Paul SM (1989) Reevaluation of the linkage relationship between chromosome 11p loci and the gene for bipolar affective disorder in the Old Order Amish. Nature 342:238–243

Kennedy JL, Guiffra LA, Moises HW, Cavalli-Sforza LL, Pakstis AJ, Kidd JR, Castiglione CM, Sjøgren B, Wetterburg L, Kid KK (1988) Evidence against linkage of schizophrenia to markers on chromosome 5 in an Northern Swedish pedigree. Nature 336:167–169

Kunkel LM, Monaco AP, Middlesworth W, Ochs HD, Latt SA (1985) Specific cloning of DNA fragments absent from the DNA of a male patient with an X chromosome deletion. Proc Natl Acad Sci USA 82:4778–4782

Lander ES, Botstein D (1986) Mapping complex genetic traits in humans: new methods using a complete RFLP linkage map. Cold Spring Harbor Symp Quant Biol 51:49–62

Mendlewicz J, Linkowski P, Wilmotte J (1980) Linkage between glucose-6-phospate dehydrogenase deficienccy and manic-depressive psychosis. Br J Psychiatry 137:337–342

Michiels F, Burmeister M, Lehrach H (1987) Derivation of clones close to met by preparative field inversion gel electrophoresis. Science 236:1305–1308

Monaco AP, Neve RL, Colletti-Feener C, Bertelson CJ, Kurnit D, Kunkel LM (1986) Isolation of candidate cDNAs for portions of the DMD gene. Nature 323:646–650

Murray R, McGuffin P, Reveley AM (1986) Genetics of schizophrenia. Psychiatr Clin North Am 9:3–16

Nakamura Y, Leppert M, O'Connell P, Wolff R, Holm T, Culver M, Martin C, Fujimoto E, Hoff M, Kumlin E, White R (1987) Variable number tandem repeat (VNTR) markers for human gene mapping. Science 235:1616–1622

Nee LE, Polinsky RJ, Eldridge R, Weingartner H, Smallberg S, Ebert M (1983) A family with histologically confirmed Alzheimer's disease. Arch Neurol 40:203–208

Oliver C, Holland AJ (1986) Down's syndrome and Alzheimer's disease: a review. Psychol Med 16:307–322

Ott J (1986) A short quide to linkage analysis. In: Davies KE (ed) Human genetic diseases, a practical approach. IRL press, Oxford UK, pp 19–32

Pericak-Vance MA, Yamaoka LH, Haynes CS, Speer MC, Haines JL, Gaskell PC, Hung W-Y, Clark CM, Heyman AL, Trfatter JA, Eisenmenger JP, Gilbert JR, Lee JE, Alberts MJ,

Dawson DV, Bartlett RJ, Earl NL, Siddique T, Vance JM, Conneally PM, Roses AD (1988) Genetic linkage studies in Alzheimer's disease families. Exp Neurol 102:271–279
Poutska AM, Lehrach H (1986) Jumping libraries and linking libraries: the next generation of molecular tools in mammalian genetics. Trends Genet 2:174–178
Poutska AM, Pohl TM, Barlow DP, Frischauf AM, Lehrach H (1987) Construction and use of human chromosome jumping libraries from NotI-digested DNA. Nature 325:353–355
Richards JE, Gilliam TC,Cole JL, Drumm ML, Wasmuth JJ, Gusella JF, Collins FS (1988) Chromosome jumping from D4S10 (G8) toward the HD gene. Proc Natl Acad Sci USA 85:6437–6441
Rommens JM, Iannuzzi MC, Kerem BS, Drumm ML, Melmer G, Dean M, Rozmahel R, Cole JL, Kennedy D, Hidaka N, Zsiga M, Buchwald M, Riordan JR, Tsui LC, Collins FS (1989) Identification of the Cystic Fibrosis gene: Chromosome walking and jumping. Science 245:1059–1065
Royer-Pokora B, Kunkel LM, Monaco AP, Goff SC, Newburger PE, Baehner RL, Sessions Cole F, Curnutte JT, Orkin SH (1986) Cloning the gene for an inherited human disorder – chronic granulomatous disease – on the basis of its chromosomal location. Nature 322:32–38
St. Clair D, Blackwood D, Muir W, Baillie D, Hubbard A, Wright A, Evans HJ (1989) No linkage of chromosome 5q11-q13 markers to schizophrenia in Scottish families. Nature 339:305–309
St. George-Hyslop PH, Tanzi RE, Polinsky RJ, Haines JL, Nee LE, Watkins PC, Myers RH, Feldman RG, Pollen D, Drachman D, Growdon J, Bruni A, Foncin J-F, Salmon D, Frommelt P, Amaducci L, Sorbi S, Piacentini S, Stewart GD, Hobbs WJ, Conneally PM, Gusella JF (1987) The genetic defect causing familial Alzheimer's disease maps on chromosome 21. Science 235:885–890
St. George-Hyslop PH, Haines JL, Farrer L, Tanzi R, Hobbs W, Polinsky RJ, Nee LE, Sorbi S, Piacentini S, Amaducci L, Heston L, Orr H, Fish S, Crapper-McLachlan D, Percy M, Frommelt P, Foncin J-F, Bruni A, Wexler N, Mayeux R, Hardy J, Goate A, Rossor M, Haynes A, James L, Owen M, Williamson R, Myers R, Feldman R, O'Sullivan D, Pollen D, O'Donnell B, Drachman D, Stowe R, Anvret M, Albo J, Sadovnick D, Growdon J, Conneally P, Gusella J (1988) Molecular genetics of autosomal dominant familial Alzheimer's disease. In: Finch CE, Davies P (eds) Current communications in molecular biology. The molecular biology of Alzheimer's disease. Cold Spring Harbor Laboratory, New York, pp 159–168
Schellenberg GD, Bird TD, Wisjman EM, Moore DK, Boehnke M, Bryant EM, Lampe TH, Nochlin D, Sumi SM, Deeb SS, Beyreuther K, Martin GM (1988) Absence of linkage of chromosome 21q21 markers to familial Alzheimer's disease. Science 241:1507–1510
Sherrington R, Brynjolfsson J, Petursson H, Potter M, Dudleston K, Barraclough B, Wasmuth J, Dobbs M, Gurling H (1988) Localisation of a susceptibility locus for schizophrenia on chromosome 5. Nature 336:164–167
Wasmuth JJ, Hewitt J, Smith B, Allard D, Haines JL, Skarecky D, Partlow E, Hayden MR (1988) A highly polymorphic locus very tightly linked to the Huntington's disease gene. Nature 332:734–736
Weber JL, May PE (1989) Abundant class of human DNA polymorphisms which can be typed using the polymerase chain reaction. Am J Hum Genet 44:388–396
Wexler NS, Bonilla E, Young AB, Shoulson J, Gomez F, Starosta S, Travers H, Villalobas M, de Quiroz I, Erke R, Penney JB, Uzzell RS, Burnham FA, Daugherty L, Jones B, Mapstone C, Rivas M, Messer E, Wexler A, Snodgrass R, Rosenzweig G, Esteves J, Marsol N, Bailey S, Bringley FJ, Goldstein E, Greene AE, Kidd JR, Kid KK, Gusella JF (1984) Huntington's disease in Venezuela and gene linkage. Cytogenet Cell Genet 37:605
White R, Lalouel JM, O'Connell P, Nakamura Y, Leppert M, Lathrop M (1987) Booklet. Genetic linkage maps for chromosomes 1, 2, 5, 6, 7, 9, 11, 12, 13, 14, 15, 16, 17, and 19. Cytogenetics and cell genetics (Human Gene Mapping 9) 46:643–649 Howard Hughes Medical Institute

Molecular Approaches Toward the Isolation of the Huntington's Disease Gene

G. Bates and *H. Lehrach*

Summary

The Huntington's disease (HD) gene has been mapped to the short arm of human chromosome 4 by genetic linkage analysis and located within the most telomeric subband 4p16.3, between the anonymous DNA marker D4S10 and the telomere. Physical mapping and cloning strategies have been used to complement genetic analysis in determining the location of the HD mutation. All available DNA markers within 4p16.3 have been used to construct a long range restriction map, consisting of three map segments together spanning 5 million base pairs (Mb) and extending minimally 4 Mb from D4S10 (the most proximal marker). Although genetic analysis is contradictory and suggests two possible positions for the gene, a telomeric location is highly probable, within 300 kilobase pairs (kb) from the end of the map. A telomere cloning vector has been constructed for the isolation and selection of human telomeres as artificial chromosomes in *Saccharomyces cerevisiae*. This has been used to clone the most distal 100 kb of the short arm of chromosone 4, confirming that the end of the long range map is the telomere and, for the first time, setting a distal limit to the position of the HD gene.

Introduction

Huntington's disease (HD) is a neurodegenerative disorder characterised by psychological disturbances, a progressive lack of motor coordination and dementia. It is inherited as an autosomal dominant disease with complete penetrance and low mutation rate. The onset of symptoms generally occurs in mid-life with progression of the disease to death over the next 15–20 years. Pathologically, the disease is characterised by the atrophy of specific classes of neurons, primarily within the striatum. The biochemistry underlying this specific cell death is unknown and there is no treatment that will arrest the course of the disease (Martin and Gusella 1986).

The HD gene was mapped to the short arm of human chromosome 4 by genetic linkage to the anonymous DNA marker D4S10 (Gusella et al. 1983) and multipoint analysis placed it distal to this marker within the most telomeric subband 4p16.3 (Gilliam et al. 1987a). The isolation of genetically linked markers has allowed the development of presymptomatic and prenatal diagnostic tests for HD (Meisson et al. 1988); however, the accuracy of such a test is compromised by a 4%

recombination frequency between D4S10 and the HD gene. Definitive testing and the potential development of a therapy will require the isolation of the defective gene and the identification of the mutation involved.

Long-range Mapping and Cloning Strategies

In the absence of chromosomal rearrangements that may indicate a novel cloning strategy, the isolation of a gene from prior knowledge of genetic linkage can be a lengthy and uncertain process. The resolution (in base pairs of DNA) associated with various mapping and cloning techniques is illustrated in Fig. 1. Genetic distances that result from linkage studies in human pedigrees are generally greater than 1 cM and approximately equivalent to millions of base pairs of DNA. The often large confidence limits associated with genetic distances can make it impossible to determine an unequivocal probe order or to position a gene with certainty

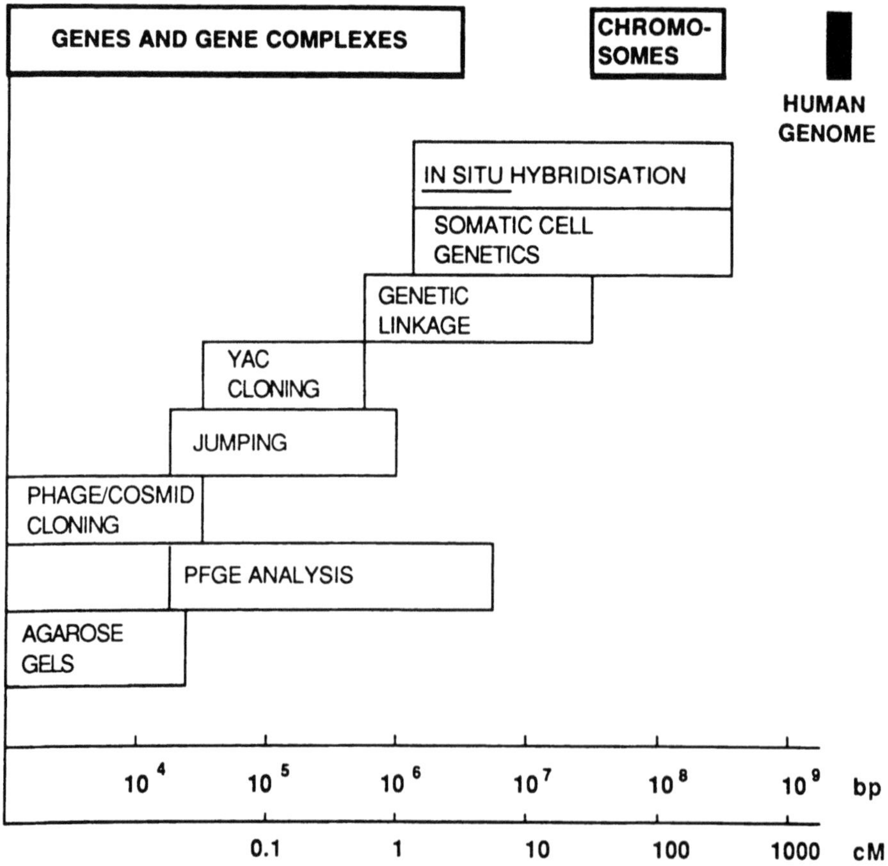

Fig. 1. The resolution in base pairs of DNA associated with available mapping and cloning strategies. The equivalent genetic distances are indicated, based on an averaged recombination frequency throughout the genome. YAC yeast artificial chromosome; PFGE pulsed field gel electrophoresis

in relation to its linked markers. In addition, the variation in recombination frequency throughout the genome makes it difficult to infer the precise physical distances between genetically linked probes. Therefore, from linkage data alone, it is not easy to determine when one is close enough to a gene to embark on the conventional cloning strategies of chromosome walking in phage or cosmid libraries, searching for conserved or expressed sequences and studying their pattern of expression to determine whether they can be implicated in the disease in question. Recently, a number of long-range physical mapping and cloning strategies have been developed that will complement genetic linkage analysis and bridge this resolution gap. These include pulsed field gel mapping, chromosome jumping and yeast artificial chromosome (YAC) libraries.

Pulsed field gel electrophoresis (PFGE) (Schwartz and Cantor 1984; Barlow and Lehrach 1987) provides the means to separate DNA fragments of up to millions of base pairs in length. Such fragments can be generated by rare cutter restriction endonucleases that detect CpG-rich recognition sequences and cut infrequently in the mammalian genome (Barlow and Lehrach 1987). Restriction maps constructed with this technology can span millions of base pairs of DNA, allowing the distances between genetically linked markers to be determined and physical limits to the position of a gene to be set. An especially useful approach is to use a specific cloning strategy (the preparation of linking libraries) to complement the restriction mapping. Linking libraries are represented by clones containing a specific rare cutter site (e.g., NotI) and probes isolated from each side of this site will, therefore, detect NotI restriction fragments that are adjacent in the genome (Poustka and Lehrach 1986).

Chromosome jumping libaries, based on the cloning of the ends of large DNA molecules, provide the technology to isolate markers hundreds of kilobases away from a starting probe in a known direction (Poustka and Lehrach 1986, 1988; Poustka et al. 1987; Collins and Weissman 1984). The construction of a jumping library with a rare cutter restriction enzyme, e.g., NotI, allows the isolation of the opposite end of a NotI fragment from a starting probe, and hence NotI jumping libraries and NotI linking libraries are complementary (Poustka and Lehrach 1986).

YAC vectors provide the ability to isolate fragments of human DNA of hundreds of kb in length as artificial chromosomes in *Saccharomyces cerevisiae* (Burke et al. 1987). These vectors not only allow the isolation of new markers, but also provide immediate access to all of the DNA within a region.

Isolation of Markers Within 4p16.3

The extreme telomeric location of the HD gene has made the search for closer and flanking markers especially difficult. Of several hundred random markers isolated from flow sorted chromosome 4 libraries, only two – D4S43 (Gilliam et al. 1987b) and D4S90 (Youngman et al. 1988) – were found to be distal to D4S10. Recently, the application of direct cloning strategies has proved to be a more fruitful approach and the construction of a number of somatic cell hybrids has greatly helped this endeavour. A hamster–human hybrid, HHW693, containing 4p15.1-

4pter translocated onto a fragment of 5p as its only human component (Wasmuth et al. 1986), has allowed access to the isolation of clones specifically in the distal half of the short arm of chromosome 4. In addition, a mapping panel has been developed that divides the 4p16.3 band into a proximal and distal portion (MacDonald et al. 1987; Smith et al. 1988).

A phage library (Smith et al. 1988; Wasmuth et al. 1988), cosmid library (Bucan et al. unpublished), and NotI linking library (Pohl et al. 1988) have been prepared from HHW693. The NotI linking library was especially productive at generating clones within the distal portion of 4p16.3, a reflection of the high denstiy of NotI sites within this region (Pohl et al. 1988). Further markers have been isolated by the end cloning of rare cutter restriction fragments from pulsed field gels (Whaley eta l. 1988) and by chromosome jumping (Pohl et al. 1988; Richards et al. 1988; Bucan et al. 1990).

A Long-range Restriction Map of 4p16.3

Pulsed field gel electrophoresis has been used to construct a long-range restriction map with more than 20 independently derived markers located within 4p16.3 (Bucan et al., 1990). The map (summarised in Fig. 2) consists of three as yet unlinked segments together covering 5 million base pairs (Mb) and extending minimally 4 Mb from D4S10 toward the telomere. The segments have been ordered and oriented by somatic cell genetics (MacDonald et al. 1987, Smith et al. 1988) and genetic linkage analysis (MacDonald et al. 1989; Youngman et al. 1989). If DNA were distributed evenly along the cytogenetic length of the chromosome, 4p16.3 should contain approximately 6 Mb, 0.2% of the human genome (Gilliam et al. 1987a). Therefore, it is likely that the majority of the DNA within 4p16.3 is

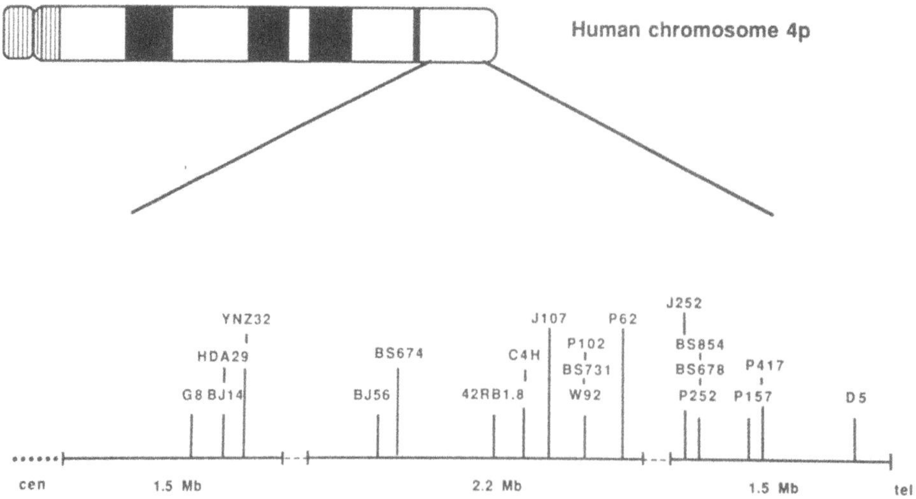

Fig. 2. A summary of the long-range restriction map of all available DNA markers genetically and physically linked to the Huntington's disease gene

represented on the map, and the gaps between the segments should not be large. The distance from the most distal marker, D5, to the end of the map is 300 kb.

Most Likely Position of the HD Gene

A number of markers used for physical mapping have been shown to display restriction fragment length polymorphisms. In many cases the recombination frequency between two markers is sufficiently low that they can be haplotyped as one locus. This is the case with C4H (D4S43) and 674 (D4S95), although they are physically separated by 700–800 kb of DNA. The genetic distances between the five haplotypes: D4S10 (G8); D4S43 (C4H)/D4S95 (BS674); D4S113 (P62)/D4S114 (P102); D4S115 (P252)/D4S111 (P157); D4S90 (D5), as determined by MacDonald et al. (1989), are illustrated in Fig. 3. Multipoint analysis indicates a map

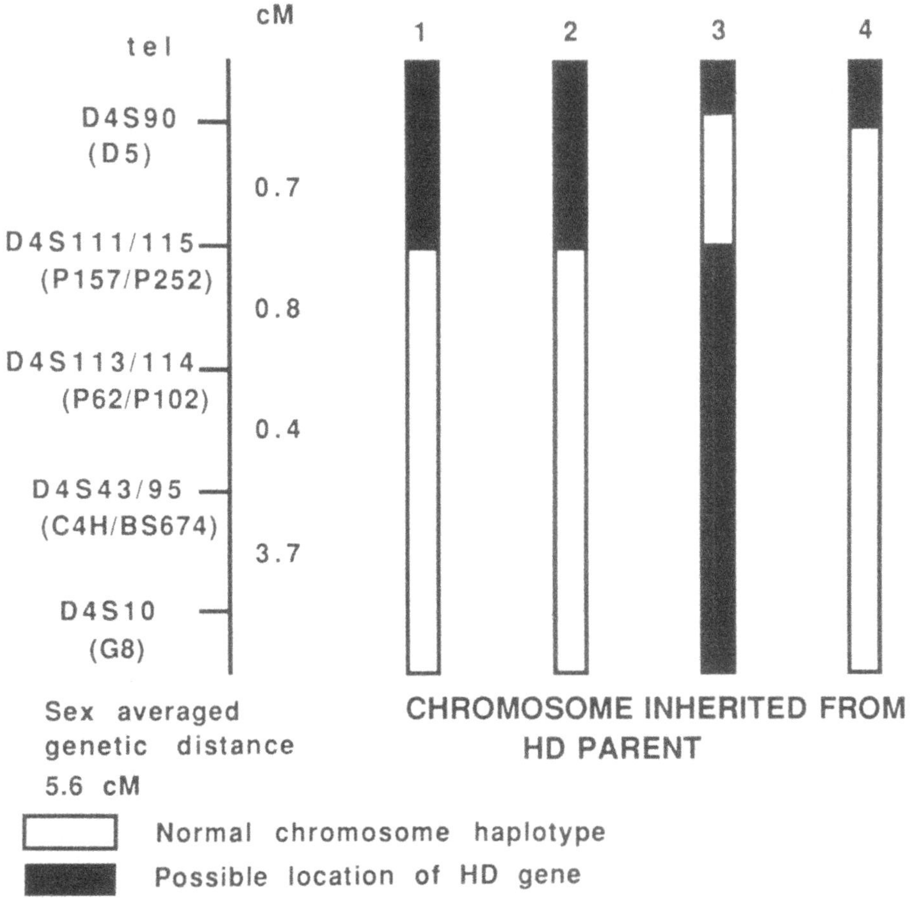

Fig. 3. A schematic summary of the genetic distances between informative markers tightly linked to the HD gene and of the most likely position of the gene, as suggested by recombination events that have been detected between these loci and the mutation. All genetic distances are sex averaged

distance of 5.6 cM between D4S10 and D4S90 (MacDonald et al. 1989; Youngman et al. 1989), more than the 3–4 cM observed for linkage between D4S10 and the HD gene, suggesting that the HD gene may be located proximal to D4S90. However, although the confidence limits are not large, the small size of the region prevents the positioning of the disease gene on the basis of comparison to the normal genetic map (MacDonald et al. 1989).

A useful strategy for pinpointing the position of a disease gene is to track informative markers through families in which a recombination event has previously been identified with the mutation. Four such recombinants have so far been reported (MacDonald et al. 1989; Robbins et al. 1989), and the results of this analysis are summarised schematically in Fig. 3. The bars represent the chromosome 4 of an affected individual that has been inherited from the parent with HD and hence must carry the HD gene. D4S90 is not informative in individuals 1 and 2, which suggests a location distal to D4S111 (MacDonald et al. 1989), but is in individual 4 (Robbins et al. 1989), placing the gene distal to D4S90. Individual 3 suggests a location proximal to D4S111/D4S115, with the D4S111/D4S115 and D4S90 loci displaying the haplotype associated with the normal chromosome. However, as this is inconsistent with the other three recombination events, the authors suggest that the most likely explanation for this observation is a double recombination event, placing the HD gene distal to D4S90 (MacDonald et al. 1989). As yet a definite flanking marker has not been detected.

Identification and Cloning of the 4p Telomere

The identification of the 4p telomere would set a distal limit to the position of the HD gene, and YAC cloning systems provide a convenient strategy for the cloning and selection of human telomeres. Conventional YAC vectors contain a yeast centromere (CEN4), a yeast replicating sequence (ARS1) and two cassettes of the telomeric repeat sequence from *Tetrahymena* (TEL) (Burke et al. 1987). The *Tetrahymena* telomeric sequences are maintained by the yeast telomerase and are functional in *Saccharomyces cerevisiae*. Telomeric repeat sequences are tandem arrays of short (6–8 bp) G–T-rich sequences, and the similarity of the human telomeric repeat to that of *Tetrahymena* (Moyzis et al. 1988) suggested that it too would be functional in yeast. A telomere cloning vector (YAC-t2) containing a single cassette of the *Tetrahymena* telomeric sequence and a rare cutter polylinker has been constructed (Fig. 4). The DNA from an individual highly likely to be homozygous for the HD gene (Wexler et al. 1987) was digested to completion with the rare cutter enzyme BssHII and used to construct a telomere library as descibed in Fig. 4.

A telomere clone containing the most distal 100 kb of chromosome 4p has been identified, derived from a chromosome carrying the HD gene in its mutant form (Bates et al. 1990). This has confirmed that the position of the telomere is at the end of the pulsed field map in Fig. 2, 300 kb from D4S90; the most distal marker on the genetic and physical maps. This has for the first time set a distal limit to the position of the HD gene and will rapidly allow the isolation of a flanking marker to the mutation.

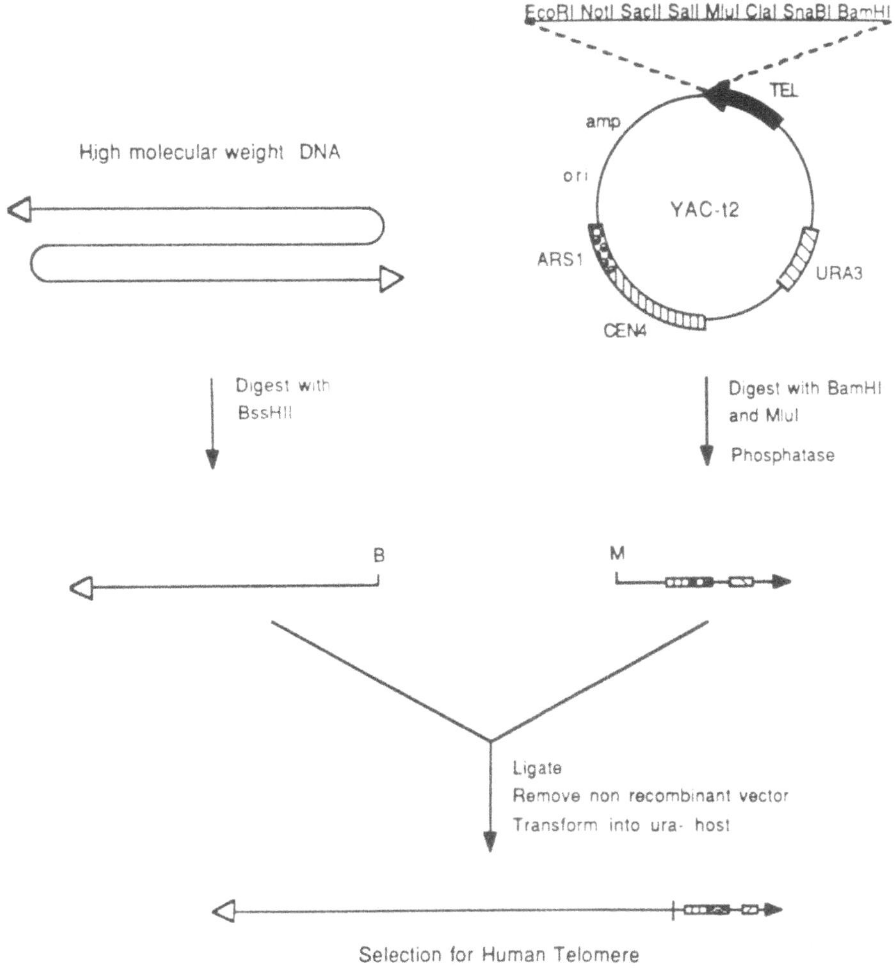

Fig. 4. Construction of a BssHII telomere library from the DNA of an individual homozygenous for the HD mutation. Cleavage of YAC-t2 with BamHI and M1uI produces a linear vector with a cassette of the *Tetrahymena* telomeric repeat sequence at one end and an M1uI cloning site at the other. Genomic DNA was cleaved to completion with BssHII and ligated to the vector (BssHII and MluI sticky ends being compatible on ligation). Transformation of the ligation reaction into ura yeast spheroplasts allowed clones derived from genomic BssHII telomeric fragments to be recovered

Acknowledgments. We wish to acknowledge our colleagues in the Hereditary Disease Foundation HD Collaborative Research Group: Charles Cantor, Francis Collins, Anna-Maria Frischauf, Jim Gusella, David Housman, Cassandra Smith, Alan Tobin and Nancy Wexler.

References

Barlow DP, Lehrach H (1987) Genetics by gel electrophoresis: the impact of pulsed field gel electrophoresis on mammalian genetics. Trends Genet 3:167–171

Bates GP, MacDonald ME, Baxendale S, Sedlacek Z, Youngman S, Romano D, Whaley WL, Alutto BA, Poustka A, Gusella JF and Lehrach H (1990) A YAC telomere clone spanning a possible location of the Huntington's disease gene. Am J Hum Genet (in press)
Bucan M, Zimmer M, Whaley WL, Poustka A, Youngman S, Allitto B, Ormondroyd E, Smith B, Pohl TM, MacDonald M, Bates GP, Richards J, Volinia S, Gilliam TC, Sedlacek Z, Collins FS, Wasmuth JJ, Shaw DJ, Gusella JF, Frischauf A-M, Lehrach H (1990). Physical maps of 4p16.3, the area expected to contain the Huntington's disease mutation. Genomics (in press)
Burke DT, Carle G, Olsen M (1987) Cloning of large segments of exogenous DNA into yeast by means of artificial chromosome vectors. Science 236:806–812
Collins FS, Weissman SM (1984) Directional cloning of DNA fragments at a large distance from an initial probe: a circularization method. Proc Natl Acad Sci USA 81:6812–6816
Gilliam TC, Tanzi RE, Haines JL, Bonner TI, Faryniarz AG, Hobbs WJ, MacDonald ME, Cheng SV, Folstein SE, Conneally PM, Wexler NS, Gusella JF (1987a) Localisation of the Huntington's disease gene to a small segment of chromosome 4 flanked by D4S10 and the telomere. Cell 50:565–571
Gilliam TC, Bucan M, MacDonald ME, Zimmer M, Haines JL, Cheng SV, Pohl TM, Meyers RH, Whaley WL, Allitto BA, Faryniarz A, Wasmuth JJ, Frischauf A-M, Conneally PM, Lehrach H, Gusella JF (1987b) A DNA segment encoding two genes very tightly linked to Huntington's disease. Science 238:950–952
Gusella JF, Wexler NS, Coneally PM, Naylor SL, Anderson MA, Tanzi RE, Watkins PC, Ottina K, Wallace MR, Sakaguchi AY, Young AB, Shoulson I, Bonilla E, Martin JB (1983) A polymorphic DNA marker genetically linked to Huntington's disease. Nature 306:234–238
MacDonald ME, Anderson MA, Gilliam TC, Tranebjaerg L, Carpenter NJ, Magenis E, Hayden MR, Healey ST, Bonner TI, Gusella JF (1987) A somatic cell hybrid panel for localising DNA segments near the Huntington's disease gene. Genomics 1:29–34
MacDonald ME, Haines JL, Zimmer M, Cheng SV, Youngman S, Whaley WL, Bucan M, Allitto BA, Smith B, Leavitt J, Poustka A, Harper P, Lehrach H, Wasmuth JJ, Frischauf A-M, Gusella JF (1989) Recombination events suggest potential sites for the Huntington's disease gene. Neuron 3:183–190
Martin JB, Gusella JF (1986) Huntington's disease: pathogenesis and management. N Engl J Med 315:1267–1276
Meisson GJ, Myers RH, Mastromauro MSW, Koroshetz WJ, Klinger KW, Farrer LA, Watkins PA, Gusella JF, Bird ED, Martin JB (1988) Predictive testing for Huntington's disease with use of a linked DNA marker. N Engl J Med 318:535–542
Moyzis RK, Buckingham JM, Cram LS, Dani M, Deaven LL, Jones MD, Meyne J, Ratcliffe RL, Wu J-R (1988) A highly conserved repetitive DNA sequence, (TTAGGG)n, present at the telomeres of human chromosomes. Proc Natl Acad Sci USA 85:6622–6626
Pohl TM, Zimmer M, MacDonald ME, Smith B, Bucan M, Poustka A, Volinia S, Searle S, Zehetner G, Wasmuth JJ, Gusella JF, Lehrach H, Frischauf A-M (1988) Construction of a NotI linking library and isolation of new markers close to the Huntington's disease gene. Nucleic Acids Res 16:9185–9189
Poustka A, Lehrach H (1986) Jumping libraries and linking libraries: the next generation of molecular tool in mammalian genetics. Trends Genet 2:174–179
Poustka A, Lehrach H (1988) Chromosome jumping: a long range cloning technique. In: Setlow JK (ed) Genetic engineering – principles and methods, vol. 10. Plenum, New York, pp 169–195
Poustka A, Pohl TM, Barlow DP, Frischauf A-M, Lehrach H (1987). Construction and use of human chromosome jumping libraries from NotI-digested DNA. Nature 325:353–355
Richards JE, Gilliam TC, Cole JL, Drumm ML, Wasmuth JJ, Gusella JF, Collins FS (1988) Chromosome jumping from D4S10 (G8) toward the Huntington's disease gene. Proc Natl Acad Sci USA 85:6437–6441
Robbins C, Theilmann J, Youngman S, Haines J, Altherr MJ, Harper PS, Payne C, Junker A, Wasmuth JJ, Hayden MR (1989) Evidence from family studies that the gene causing Huntington's disease is telomeric to D4S95 and D4S90. Am J Hum Genet 44:422–425
Schwartz DC, Cantor CR (1984) Separation of yeast chromosome-sized DNAs by pulsed field gradient gel electrophoresis. Cell 37:67–75

Smith B, Skarecky D, Bengtsson U, Magenis RE, Carpenter N, Wasmuth JJ (1988) Isolation of DNA markers in the direction of the Huntington's disease gene from the G8 locus. Am J Hum Genet 42:335–344

Wasmuth JJ, Carlock LR, Smith B, Immken LL (1986) A cell hybrid and recombinant DNA library that facilitate identification of polymorphic loci in the vicinity of the Huntington disease gene. Am J Hum Genet 39:397–403

Wasmuth JJ, Hewitt J, Smith B, Allard D, Haines JL, Skarecky D, Partlow E, Hayden MR (1988) A highly polymorphic locus very tightly linked to the Huntington's disease gene. Nature 322:734–736

Wexler NS, Young, AB, Tanzi RE, Travers H, Starosta-Rubinstein S, Penney JB, Snodgrass SR, Shoulson I, Gomez F, Ramos Arroyo MA, Penchaszadeh GK, Moreno H, Gibbons K, Faryniarz A, Hobbs W, Anderson MA, Bonilla E, Conneally PM, Gusella GF (1987) Homozygotes for Huntington's disease. Nature 326:194–197

Whaley WL, Michiels F, MacDonald ME, Romano D, Zimmer M, Smith B, Leavitt J, Bucan M, Haines JL, Gilliam TC, Zehetner G, Smith C, Cantor CR, Frischauf A-M, Wasmuth JJ, Lehrach H, Gusella JF (1988) Mapping of D4S98/S114/S113 confines the Huntington's defect to a reduced physical region at the telomere of chromosome. 4. Nucleic Acids Res 16:11769–11780

Youngman S, Shaw DJ, Gusella JF, MacDonald ME, Stanbridge EJ, Wasmuth JJ, Harper PS (1988) A DNA probe, D5 (D4S90) mapping to human chromosome 4p16.3. Nucleic Acids Res 16:1648

Youngman S, Sarfarazi M, Bucan M, MacDonald ME, Smith B, Zimmer M, Gilliam TC, Frischauf A-M, Wasmuth JJ, Gusella JF, Lehrach H, Harper PS, Shaw DJ (1989) A new DNA marker (D4S90) is terminally located on the short arm of chromosome 4, close to the Huntington's disease gene. Genomics 5:802–809

Impact of Environmental Mutagens on Mental Health

R. J. Šrám, B. Binková and *J. A. Gebhart*

Summary

The effects of mutagens have been seen in the increase of birth defects in the general population as well as in children whose parents were exposed to mutagens in the workplace. Due to the well-known fact that at least half of genes are related to the mental functions, behavioural changes resulting from exposure to mutagens should be expected. There are three important areas of interest:
a) alcohol;
b) drugs, combined with environmental pollution, and
c) the effect of antioxidants which may suppress free radical action in aging.

The effects of environmental mutagens on behavioural changes should be studied to determine whether mutagens in polluted regions may also increase neuro-psycho-behavioural abnormalities in local populations and, in the long run, impair the mental health of society as a whole.

Introduction

Chemical, physical and biological mutagens induce DNA changes, which are expressed during the next cell divisions as the changed genetic information. The functional change of the mutated gene is phenotypically manifested as the genetic injury. Environmental mutagens may damage DNA through direct interaction or indirectly, through their metabolites. Both can affect the process of DNA repair (inhibition of enzymes) or induce free radicals. The impact of the mutations is related to the type of injured cells. Mutations induced in gametes increase the frequency of spontaneous abortions, birth defects, inborn errors of metabolism, predisposition to faster aging and cancer, as well as brain maldevelopment and deficient repair of genetic damage. Mutations in somatic cells correspond to teratogeny in the fetus; in an adult organism they speed up aging, change neuronal transmission and increase the risk of cancer.

In evaluating the genetic risk of mutagens, it should be clear that each human phenotype is the result of interaction between the genotype and the environment. The impact on an individual of each environmental mutagen, even before it acts in his or her DNA, may be exacerbated by other factors, e.g., stress, drugs, alcohol, smoking or occupational exposure to mutagens.

Present knowledge indicates the significance of oxidative damage to the human organism and the connection between lipid peroxidation (LPO) and the DNA repair mechanism as process which may speed up the aging process as well as the course of several diseases (e.g., cancer, atherosclerosis, hypertension, Alzheimer's disease). The current theory about the relationship between the induction of free oxygen radicals and these damaging actions presupposes an increase of LPO and a decrease in DNA repair capacity. This theory is also supported by the idea that oxidative damage may be suppressed by antioxidants acting as free radical scavengers (Šrám et al. 1986).

To determine whether these theoretical assumptions represent a real risk for humans the theory was tested between 1982 and 1986 in a study of the frequency of birth defects in three districts in Czechoslovakia with different types of environmental pollution. District A is polluted by soft-coal power stations, mines, and the chemical industry; district B by soft-coal power stations and mines; and district C by soft-coal power stations from regions outside the district. There were increased concentrations of sulphur dioxide and nitrogen oxides in all three regions. A total of 18 060 pregnancies were studied. The average frequency of birth defects observed in each district was: A 9.8%; B 8.7%, and C 6.4%. When the effects of longlasting smog caused by inversions (such as seen in district A in the winter of 1982, which lasted for several weeks) were compared with the conception and early stages of pregnancy of the group of children conceived in this period, it was noted that the frequency of birth defects increased by at least 50%.

Evaluating the mutagenic and teratogenic effects of occupational exposure in these regions, we observed several high risk groups (Table 1; Bochkov and Šrám 1989). These data indicated that mutagens in our environment could increase birth defects in the general population as well as among children whose parents were exposed to mutagens in the workplace.

Man has 50000–100000 structural genes that encode the nucleotide sequence of various RNAs and the amino acid structure of proteins. It has been estimated that

Table 1. Birth defects and parents' occupational exposure

Exposure to	Group	No. of examined children	Frequency compared with unexposed group (%)
Mothers	Total	8235	
	Chemical industry	93	+73
	Hairdressing	32	+34
	Hospitals	317	+33
	Agriculture	162	+26
	Mines	82	+23
Fathers	Total	7695	
	Chemical industry	130	+52
	Mines	412	+44
	Painting	75	+24
	Hospitals	94	+23
	Agriculture	315	+19
	Glassworks	275	+14

approximately 50% of structural genes affect the mental functions and at least one third of genetic diseases are manifested in the central nervous system. Behavioral changes resulting from the impact of mutagens should be expected. Most vulnerable may be perinatal brain development, which is characterised by intensive histogenesis and cytodifferentiation.

The possible effects of mutagens on mental functions, expressed as behavioral changes, have not been studied sufficiently. The reason may be the lack of epidemiological studies that indicate that mutagens may be the real problem, at least for some countries. In fact, until recently no negative effects of mutagens on behaviour were observed. These problems may be very important in the future. Therefore, the World Health Organization should encourage studies in three areas of interest:

a) alcohol;
b) drugs, and their effects in combination with pollution; and
c) the effect of antioxidants on aging.

Alcohol

The genetic risk of chronic alcoholism may be related to the mutagenic and carcinogenic activity of acetaldehyde (AA). The ability of AA to cause LPO has been linked to AA oxidation and glutathione reduction. AA has also been found to impair the repair of alkylated nucleoproteins (Obe and Anderson 1987).

In analysing the effect of alcohol abuse on unscheduled DNA synthesis (UDS, which gives information about the efficiency of excision repair), LPO and levels of vitamins (Table 2), we observed a significant decrease of UDS and vitamins C and B_{12}, as well as an increase of LPO in plasma and lymphocytes (Šrám et al. 1989). Comparing the most sensitive parameters (UDS and LPO) between groups of chronic alcoholics and elderly males, it appears that chronic alcohol consumption speeds up the process of aging by at least 15 years, if we accept UDS and LPO levels as indicators of aging (Table 3). These results show that abstinence alone is

Table 2. Effects of alcohol abuse on UDS, LPO and vitamin levels in men (± s.d.)

Group	Alcoholics	Controls
Number	62	33
Age (years)	39.9 ± 9.3	39.0 ± 9.8
UDS (T/C)	3.65 ± 0.59[a]	4.73 ± 0.98
LPO plasma (nmol MDA/ml)	1.47 ± 0.49[a]	1.09 ± 0.26
LPO lymphocytes (nmol/mg)	1.79 ± 0.61[a]	1.23 ± 0.31
Ascorbic acid (mg/l)	4.9 ± 3.5[a]	12.2 ± 4.9
α-Tocopherol (mg/l)	10.3 ± 3.1	9.8 ± 3.2
Retinol (mg/l)	0.72 ± 0.19	0.70 ± 0.19
Vitamin B_{12} (ng/l)	231 ± 175[a]	538 ± 250

[a] $P < 0.001$

T-lymphocytes treated with alkylating agent MNNG, C-control samples, T/C – the level of incorporation of (^{3}H)thymidine as the consequence of the DNA damage by MNNG (excision repair)

Table 3. Effects of age and alcohol abuse on UDS and LPO levels in men (± s.d.)

Group	Alcoholics	Elderly males			Controls
Age (years)	38.4	60–69	70–79	>80	37.9
Number	52	9	20	20	23
UDS (T/C)	3.77 ± 0.60	3.48 ± 0.62	3.41 ± 0.77	2.94 ± 0.77	4.72 ± 0.59
LPO plasma (nmol MDA/ml)	1.55 ± 0.14	1.38 ± 0.30	1.33 ± 0.26	1.41 ± 0.35	1.12 ± 0.14
LPO lymphocytes (nmol MDA/mg)	1.79 ± 0.29	1.60 ± 0.51	1.47 ± 0.28	1.43 ± 0.34	1.14 ± 0.19

not sufficient to improve all injury caused by the long-term overconsumption of alcohol.

Drugs

Experimental studies as well as clinical screenings indicate that some drugs and diet deficiency may be responsible for the impaired brain functions expressed as neuro-psycho-behavioural abnormalities, usually referred to as minimal brain dysfunction (MBD – the hyperkinetic child, emotional lability with impulsive and aggressive acts, impaired motor coordination, specific learning disabilities such as dyslexia).

Recently the frequency of birth defects has increased in several regions of Czechoslovakia. Simultaneously, there has been observed an increased number of children who are not able to pass the first class in primary school due to neurobehavioural problems. Behavioural teratology studies in rats stimulated the idea that nootropics might ameliorate the brain injury and later clinical studies demonstrated that nootropics did ameliorate MBD, if they were administered in time. The same methods can be used to study unfavourable effects of new drugs applied in the period of perinatal brain development (Benešová et al. 1984).

Nevertheless, the extrapolation of experimental results from animals to humans may be questionable as shown in recent results from mutagenicity studies with paracetamol (PC). This drug is widely used as an analgesic and antipyretic, especially in children and pregnant women. It was believed that no side effects could be expected. However, studies on human volunteers, using a dose of $3 \times 1\,000$ mg administered over an 8-h period, found an increase of chromosome aberrations in peripheral lymphocytes and suppression of UDS (Table 4); Kočišová et al. 1988; Topinka et al. 1989). It may be expected that PC would affect brain development similarly. As the genotoxicity of PC was not observed at the mammalian level, the lesson should be that mutagenicity studies should also be done on human volunteers when testing a new drug in phase I of a clinical trial.

Special care should be given to the evaluation of the genetic risk of drugs in highly polluted regions. For example as sulphur dioxide suppresses the repair of genetic damage, it may be that drug with mutagenic effects may cause more serious injury in regions with high sulphur dioxide levels. This may be particularly

Table 4. Paracetamol cytogenetic analysis and UDS in human peripheral lymphocytes (N = 11)

Time (h) after first dose	AB.C. (%)	UDS (T/C)
0	1.68 ± 0.30	5.02 ± 0.47
24	2.77 ± 0.36[a]	4.11 ± 0.56[b]
72	2.14 ± 0.27	4.46 ± 0.66
168	1.45 ± 0.42	5.07 ± 0.37

[a] $P < 0.05$
[b] $P < 0.01$

important for example, in the treatment of schizophrenics. Long-term therapy by neuroleptics increases the frequency of chromosome aberrations in peripheral lymphocytes (aberrant cells, AB.C.) and LPO in plasma, and decreases UDS (Table 5; Šrám et al. 1989).

Effects of Antioxidants on Aging

Recombinant DNA techniques indicate that the gene for Alzheimer's disease is located on chromosome 21, linked to the gene for superoxide dismutase (SOD). This finding encourages a stimulating approach, relating Alzheimer's disease to free radical action.

The hypothesis generated by this approach is that, if we are able to diagnose Alzheimer's disease, we might use this knowledge to advise the proband to change his or her lifestyle (diet, stress) and thereby to postpone the first signs of disease for several months or years. Because the effect of free radicals may be suppressed by antioxidants, the first choice of treatment could be natural antioxidants, such as α-tocopherol and ascorbic acid.

Nevertheless, this approach simultaneously hides an ethical problem. Is it correct to use recombinant DNA techniques, diagnose Alzheimer's disease and start antioxidant supplementations, thereby burdening the patient with the knowledge of the disease?

Table 5. Effects of neuroleptics on chromosome aberrations, UDS and LPO levels in schizophrenics (± s.d.)

Group	Schizophrenics	Controls
Number	24	23
Age (years)	48.1 ± 11.8	38.3 ± 6.0
Analyses cells	2400	2300
AB.C. (%)	2.60	1.52
B/C	0.037	0.016
UDS (T/C)	2.95 ± 0.91[a]	3.63 ± 0.85
LPO plasma (nmolk MDA/ml)	1.41 ± 0.22[b]	1.09 ± 0.13
Ascorbic acid (mg/l)	5.3 ± 3.5	10.1 ± 3.6

[a] $P < 0.05$
[b] $P < 0.01$

Table 6. Effects of 12-month antioxidant supplementation on UDS, LPO and vitamin levels in an elderly population (± s.d.)

	Males		Females	
Antioxidants	–	+	–	+
Number	21	32	54	26
Age (years)	73.4 ± 9.7	74.3 ± 10.2	80.2 ± 8.2	78.6 ± 8.6
UDS (T/C)	3.91 ± 0.85	4.11 ± 0.64	3.74 ± 0.85	3.92 ± 0.68
LPO plasma (nmol MDA/ml)	1.55 ± 0.22	1.35 ± 0.21[b]	1.54 ± 0.26	1.37 ± 0.21[b]
LPO lymphocytes (nmol MDA/mg)	1.68 ± 0.21	1.45 ± 0.21[c]	1.61 ± 0.32	1.42 ± 0.24
Ascorbic acid (mg/l)	2.2 ± 1.9	17.8 ± 4.6[c]	3.6 ± 2.4	18.1 ± 5.2[c]
α-Tocopherol (mg/l)	7.6 ± 3.2	13.4 ± 4.9[a]	9.5 ± 3.4	18.1 ± 8.7[a]
Retinol (mg/l)	0.47 ± 0.28	0.59 ± 0.18	0.63 ± 0.19	0.59 ± 0.17
Vitamin B_{12} (ng/l)	207 ± 184	187 ± 266	169 ± 146	199 ± 218

[a] $P < 0.05$
[b] $P < 0.01$
[c] $P < 0.005$

The effects of antioxidants on the process were studied on an elderly population from rest homes who were given supplements of a daily dose of 300 mg α-tocopherol and 1 000 mg ascorbic acid for 1 year. The most significant changes were observed in LPO levels in plasma and lymphocytes (Table 6). Psychological tests were used to determine verbal and numerical memory, drawing sensomotor reactivity, subjective feelings and the Crichton test, from which the depression

Table 7. Effects of 12-month antioxidant supplementation on psychological tests in an elderly population (± s.d.)

	Males		Females	
Antioxidants	+	–	+	–
Numerical memory				
I	4.79 ± 1.15[b]	3.80 ± 0.63	4.51 ± 1.00[a]	3.89 ± 1.25
N	34	10	33	27
II	2.47 ± 1.11[b]	1.22 ± 1.20	2.29 ± 1.16[b]	1.22 ± 1.34
N	34	9	31	27
Verbal memory	6.73 ± 2.15	5.70 ± 2.75	7.77 ± 2.26[c]	4.55 ± 2.46
N	33	10	31	22
Drawing	3.95 ± 2.36[c]	1.15 ± 1.81	4.03 ± 2.42[c]	1.03 ± 2.36
N	38	20	39	33
Subjective Feeling	39.1 ± 20.2	34.0 ± 23.1	50.2 ± 19.1	55.3 ± 19.3
N	35	10	30	23
Crichton	30.6 ± 8.0[b]	34.7 ± 10.4	32.3 ± 9.7[b]	35.2 ± 9.8
N	122	61	161	184
Depression score	6.15 ± 1.43[b]	7.15 ± 2.12	6.31 ± 1.64[c]	7.07 ± 1.96
N	122	61	161	184

[a] $P < 0.05$
[b] $P < 0.01$
[c] $P < 0.001$

score was calculated separately. The antioxidant supplementation significantly improved numerical memory in males and females and verbal memory in females, as well as the results of the Crichton test (Table 7). This indicates that long-term antioxidant supplementation may improve cognitive functions (Šrám et al. 1989).

These results seem to indicate that long-term antioxidants supplementation, lasting for more than 6 months, may decrease the LPO process in the aging organism and thereby decrease the DNA damage induced by free radicals.

Conclusion

Summing up our results we may conclude that long- lasting antioxidant supplementation suppresses the damaging effect of oxygen radicals on DNA, proteins and biomembranes in the aging process and in other free radical diseases, such chronic alcoholism and schizophrenia.

It would be useful to support studies on the effects of mutagens on behavioral changes to learn if the mutagens in polluted regions may also increase neuro-psycho-behavioural abnormalities in local populations and in the long run, impair the mental health of society as a whole.

References

Benešová O, Pavlik A, Pětová J (1984) Brain maldevelopment and drugs. Avicenum, Prague

Bochkov NP, Šrám RJ (1989) Modern trends and realities of genetic monitoring. Biol Zentalbl 108:341–348

Kočišová J, Rossner P, Binková B, Bavorová H, Šrám RJ (1988) Mutagenicity studies of paracetamol in human volunteers. I. Cytogenetic analysis of peripheral lymphocytes and lipid peroxidation in plasma. Mutat Res 209:161–165

Obe A, Anderson D (1987) Genetic effects of ethanol. Mutat Res 186:177–200

Šrám J, Binková B, Kočišová J, Topinka J, Fojtiková I, Hanel I, Klaschka J, Kotěšovec F, Gebhart JA (1989) Antioxidants effect on alcohol, drugs and aging. Liss, New York (in press)

Šrám RJ, Černá M, Holá N (1986) Effect of ascorbic acid prophylaxis in groups occupationally exposed to mutagens. In: Ramel C, Lambert B, Magnusson J (eds) Genetic effects and applied mutagenesis. Liss, New York, pp 327–335

Topinka J, Šrám J, Širinjan G, Kočišová J, Binková B, Fojtíková I (1989) Mutagenicity studies on paracetamol in human volunteers. II. Unscheduled DNA synthesis and micronucleous test. Mutat Res 227:147–152

Development of an Infrastructure for Molecular Genetic Analysis in Psychiatry

M. Smith and *S. Potkin*

Clinical Material

Molecular genetic studies in psychiatry are dependent upon the development of repositories of clinical information and genetic material derived from a large number of families in which there are family members with clinically and biologically characterized psychiatric illness. It seems likely that major psychiatric illness is caused by a series of different genes which may exert their effects singly or, in some instances, together. It is therefore particularly important that material be obtained from a large number of families to address questions of genetic heterogeneity. Ideally, families for genetic studies should be derived from population groups from various parts of the world, since the various genes involved in determining susceptibility to development of psychiatric illness may have different frequencies in different populations.

Family Size and Structure

Although much progress has been made in genetic linkage analysis through the utilization of large pedigrees in which a particular genetic disease occurs in a large number of individuals, for example, Huntington's chorea (Gusella et al. 1983), it is important to be aware that, if only high-density families are utilized, we may in the case of certain diseases be selecting for particular subtypes of an illness. If small families are utilized, perhaps the minimum informative structure is an affected proband with one unaffected sib and both parents available.

Diagnostic Criteria

Ideally, a number of different classification systems should be used for defining psychiatric illness in families to be included in genetic linkage studies. It is critically important that comprehensive descriptions be available regarding the classification systems and thresholds used.

Development of Comprehensive Data Bases

Progress in delineating the molecular basis of psychiatric illness will be expedited by the development of comprehensive data bases which include not only clinical diagnostic information and results of genetic marker analysis but also neurophysiological, neuroendocrine, and neurochemical indices and neuropharmacological information.

Aspects of linkage Analysis

In carrying out linkage analysis in psychiatric illness it will most likely be important to utilize models based on several different modes of inheritance and various different degrees of penetrance. Particular emphasis may need to be placed on affected individuals within one family. Since the development of overt psychiatric disease may require the predisposing gene and additional factors (e.g., age-related factors, inducers), unaffected family members may provide less information. Ongoing exchange of ideas between clinicians and statisticians will be valuable to devise better models for linkage analysis in psychiatric illness.

Studies in Special Populations

There are a number of examples in the literature in which mapping of genetic disease genes was greatly facilitated by the identification of individuals in whom genetic disease was cosegregating with a cytogenetically detectable structural chromosomal aberration. One example of this is the deletion on the X chromosome which facilitated mapping of the Duchenne muscular dystrophy disease gene (Franke et al. 1985). Detection in particular families of the cosegregation of psychiatric illness and chromosomal rearrangements could greatly facilitate identification of chromosomal regions which are important in the causation of such illnesses.

It is therefore important to obtain a careful family history to identify those families with mental illness and a history of multiple miscarriages or developmental abnormalities present in immediate or extended family. If such families are identified, chromosome analyses should be carried to search, for example, for balanced and unbalanced chromosome translocation carriers.

Collection and Handling of Samples

Wherever possible, efforts should be made to obtain blood samples suitable for establishing lymphoblastoid cell lines. Such cell lines not only serve as a resource for preparation of DNA but can be utilized subsequently for analysis of large fragments of DNA, e.g., utilizing pulse-field gel electrophoresis.

In situations in which it is not possible to establish cell lines, alternate procedures may be used, e.g., obtaining white blood cell samples for DNA preparation, freezing of white blood cells or whole blood in DMSO for subsequent culture, or freezing of white cells for subsequent DNA isolation. In collecting samples for linkage analysis it is important to store red cells and plasma/serum since protein markers may be valuable.

Possibilities for Various Centers to Participate in Different Phases of Molecular Genetic Analyses in Psychiatric Disorders

In establishing an infrastructure for molecular genetic studies in psychiatry it is important to note that there are different phases of the projects, including clinical evaluation, laboratory analyses, and statistical analyses.

Centers may participate in one or more of the following phases:

1. Identification of families and patient groups of interest.
2. Obtaining blood samples for storage or for establishing cell lines. In phases 1 and 2 investigators will need to be aware of sociocultural factors which may affect the obtaining of information about family structure or obtaining blood samples.
3. Karyotypic analysis in special groups of patients.
4. Analysis of polymorphic DNA markers. Centers involved in such studies will need to have available a large series of informative polymorphic DNA probes.
5. Linkage analysis. Centers involved in linkage analysis will need to have available programs for two-point and multipoint linkage analysis and facilities for maintaining comprehensive data bases for information gathered in families submitted for linkage analysis.
6. Derivation of new probes in specific chromosomal regions which appear to be important in psychiatric illness, based on the results of linkage analyses.
7. Analysis of large fragments of DNA through pulse-field gel or CHEF gel electrophoresis to define the presence, at a molecular genetic level, of possible deletions or rearrangements.
8. mRNA analysis. Having identified chromosomal regions which are closely linked to specific psychiatric disorders, it will be advantageous to have available tissue banks containing brain tissue, so that mRNA can be prepared and subsequently screened for detection of expressed sequences.
9. Analysis of DNA sequence.

References

Francke U, Ochs HD, de Martinville B, Giacalone J, Lindgren V, Disteche C, Pagon RA, Hofker MH, van Ommen GKB, Pearson PL, Wedgwood RJ (1985) Minor Xp21 chromosome deletion in a male associated with expression of Duchenne muscular dystrophy, chronic granulomatous disease, retinitis pigmentosa, and McLeod syndrome. Am J Hum Genet 37:250

Gusella JF, Wexler NS,Coneally PM, Naylor S, Anderson MA, Tanzi RE, Watkins PC, Ottina K, Wallace M, Sakaguchi A, Young A, Shoulson I,Bonilla E, Martin JB (1983) A polymorphic DNA marker genetically linked to Huntington's disease. Nature 306:234–238

Status of Human Genetics and Genetic Psychiatric Research in India

S. S. Agarwal and *B. B. Sethi*

At the outset it is necessary to state that the account that follows is a personal perspective. In this review an attempt is made only to focus on those major areas of human genetics which have been either studied or need to be studied in the Indian context. It is neither intended nor possible to be comprehensive in this brief narration.

Indirect suggestions indicate that the role of hereditary factors was appreciated by our ancient men of knowledge. For example, the importance of quality of sperms and the mother's health in determining the outcome of the pregnancy and the health of the offspring is indicated in the Rigveda (Anonymous). Also, counselling regarding preselection of sex and conduct during pregnancy to avoid congenital anomalies have been practised as part of the Ayurvedic system of medicine for several centuries (Charak Samhita 1941). Furthermore, the marital laws prohibited marriages among relations up to seven generations.

In recent times, the importance of genetic heterogeneity among Indian populations was recognised by Haldane in the 1950s. He chose India as his last home and stimulated a group of young investigators to study genes in the population (Crow 1985). This led to several studies on genetic markers in both tribal and nontribal groups in different parts of the country (Satyawaki 1983, Mourant et al. 1984; Bhatia and Rao 1986). One of the outcomes of these studies has been the recognition of the high prevalence of sickle cell anaemia, thalassemia and G-6-PD deficiency in several tribal populations in India (Bhatia and Rao 1986). However, the impact of these disorders on tribal health is still not fully appreciated and the provision of medical care to deal with these medical problems remains to be upgraded. An effort in this direction has been made by the Indian Council of Medical Research (ICMR) through its Regional Medical Research Centres at Jabalpur, Dibrugarh and Bhuvneshwar. The ICMR Institute of Immunohaematology at Bombay, the National Institute of Health and Family Welfare, New Delhi, and several other individual investigators are also actively engaged in this field.

In addition, population genetic studies have helped in consolidating the historical and anthropometric data indicating the existence of three major racial groups in the Indian population, i.e., Caucasoids in North-Western India, Mongoloids in North Eastern India and Dravidians in South India (Mayumbar 1961). The gene frequencies of several genetic markers have been reported to be quite distinct for these population groups, but the biological significance of these differences is not explored. Most of these studies have been carried out at the "macro" level, i.e., comparing tribal with nontribal populations, North Indians with South Indians,

Hindus with Muslims etc. In some instances caste groups have also been studied. But to the best of our knowledge, population genetic studies have not been carried out in discrete homogeneous population samples at the "micro" level, which is more likely to demonstrate genetically determined differences compared with larger, heterogeneous groups. One can cite the example of Indian childhood cirrhosis, a disease peculiar to Indian subcontinent, which occurs predominantly in Vaish and Brahmin communities of Hindus (Liver Disease Sub-committee of ICMR 1955; Agarwal et al. 1979). Another recent example is of a peculiar spondyloepiphyseal skeletal dysplasia which occurs almost exclusively in Harijans, a group of Hindus, in a localised pocket in South India (unpublished observations). Likewise, a high prevalence of diabetes has been reported in Patels from Gujrat who have settled in Great Britain (Mather and Keen 1985) and coronary artery disease in settlers of Indian origin in the Caribean (Beckles et al. 1986). It has to be recognised that peculiar sociocultural practices and marital patterns might have created a variety of genetic subsets in Indian society (Bala Krishan 1978). There are four major religions in India, i.e., Hindu, Muslim, Sikh and Christian. Among Hindus there are four major castes, i.e., Kshatriya, Brahmin, Vaish and Harijans, and within each caste there are several subcastes. Generally marriages among Hindus are in the same caste and restricted to a limited region. In a few selected instances endogamy is practiced even at the subcaste level, e.g., among Chaturvedis, Mathurs, Bhargavas and Rastogies at Lucknow it is common practice to marry within the same subcaste (surname/last name), though there is no consanguinity as far as one can trace the history through living relatives. Theoretically, long-standing endogamy could lead to genetic differentiation which can influence the susceptibility to multifactorial diseases. Whether or not it happens remains to be studied; until such time it is prudent to control for this variable in genetic epidemiological studies.

For testing of genetic heterogeneity at the micro level, HLA polymorphism and restriction fragment length polymorphism (RFLP) are expected to be more useful. In a study using HLA polymorphism, Pitchappan (1988) from Madurai has shown significant differences in haplotype frequencies in different caste groups from the same geographic area. Our observations comparing HLA haplotype frequencies among Hindus at Lucknow (unpublished observations) with those at Delhi (Mehra et al. 1986) also show that Hindus of North India are a heterogeneous group.

Also influential in human genetic research in India has been Dr. Khanolkar. Perhaps impressed by the observation of a high prevalence of mammary cancer in Parsee women in India, he set up a genetic unit at Cancer Research Institute, Bombay, in the 1950s. The group identified a very high prevalence of G-6-PD deficiency in Parsees (up to 20%), but the factors which might influence the aggregation of breast cancer in this population still remain elusive (Jussawala et al. 1981). This group led by Dr. Sanghvi at CRI also became interested in the genetic consequences of the high prevalence of consanguinity in Hindus of South India. However, contrary to expectations, they did not find any significant difference in reproductive performances between consanguineous and nonconsanguineous couples (Sanghvi 1966). This has led them to hypothesise that long-standing consanguinity has wiped out the deleterious genes from the population. Likewise, Rao and

Inbaraj (1971, 1983, 1987) did not find any significant effect of consanguinity on total foetal loss rates, neonatal, infant, perinatal and extended first-year mortality rates, or fertility and sterility rates. In more recent studies Appaji Rao's group at Bangalore (Radha Rami Devi et al. 1987) also did not find any significant difference in the prevalence of single gene determined amino acid disorders between consanguineous and non-consanguineous groups.

Whether this is a limitation of methodology or a true biological phenomenon remains to be seen. Theoretically, consanguinity should lead to homozygosity at recessive loci. One should measure homozygosity at HLA and RFLP loci which are known to be extremely polymorphic. Also, one would need to separate out the causes of childhood mortality in the population as well as study for late effects. High infant mortality rates may mask expression of genetic disorders. Interestingly, in North India there is no consanguinity in Hindus. However, among Muslims in North India the consanguinity rate may be as high as in Hindus in the South (Basu 1975). This may be another group which can be studied for the effects of consanguinity. From the foregoing it can be concluded that, for genetic epidemiological studies in the Indian context, race, religion and consanguinity must be closely matched.

Very soon after the discovery of the correct number of human chromosomes, Indian scientists became interested in cytogenetics. The lead was taken by university departments of botany, zoology and anthropology. Later, cytogenetics was taken up by departments of anatomy in medical schools and they were responsible for the introduction of some human genetics in the medical curriculum. At present there are more than 50 active human cytogenetic laboratories in the country. Many of these are associated with clinical genetic services providing diagnostic service to patients. Besides, these laboratories are engaged in evaluation of chromosomal aberrations and sister chromatid exchange (SCE) frequencies in populations exposed to potential mutagenic/teratogenic agents. Lately in situ hybridisation techniques have been introduced at some centres in India and molecular cytogenetics is developing. Some groups have also set up facilities for amniotic fluid fibroblast cultures and chorionic villus sampling, but antenatal diagnosis of cytogenetic disorders is not yet routine.

Recognising the importance of genetic disorders to maternal child health and the need to augment genetic services in the context of population control strategies, the ICMR has provided sustained support to clinical genetic research during the past 7–8 years. The tragedy of Bhopal, where more than 2 000 lives were lost following accidental leakage of MIC gas, has further heightened the awareness of genetic problems. There are about a dozen active clinical genetic centres in the country at present. In addition to participating in the documentation of the prevalence of genetic disorders, these centres are also focusing on the development of counselling and prenatal diagnostic facilities. Many of these centres are located in large cities in different parts of the country (Bombay, Bangalore, Calcutta, Hyderabad, Lucknow, Madras, New Delhi, Pune, etc.), which in due course may emerge as regional genetic centres.

The impact of clinical genetics on the practice of medicine in India has been rather limited so far. One of the main activities of those interested in this field has been the study of the prevalence of congenital malformations in different geographic areas (Verma and Mathews 1983). It has been found that open neural tube defects (NTD) is the most common congenital malformation. The highest prevalence of NTD has been reported in Sikhs from Punjab (5–8/1 000) and the trait has been reported to exhibit from gradient from west to east and north to south tread (Verma 1978). However, in spite of long-term interest in congenital malformations, the facilities for accurate diagnosis of prenatal and perinatal disease is not yet adequate and counselling is usually empirical. There is no active congenital malformation registry in the country to the best of our knowledge. Most of the studies on congenital malformations have been carried out at medical School based referal hospitals. The history of drug intake, including self-medication in the first trimester, was found to have significant association with occurence of congenital malformations, but exact information about suspected drugs agents is not available (unpublished observations). This includes the use of Ayurvedic and homeopathic medicines as well, the systems which are widely practiced in India.

The development of biochemical and molecular human genetics in India has not kept pace with other nations. The reason may be that the practice of medicine in India is still very much preoccupied with infections. Diarrhoea and respiratory tract infections remain the major causes of infant and childhood mortality.

Most of the medical schools do not teach medical genetics. There is hardly any exposure of medical students to the scope of modern molecular medicine. However, the situation is likely to change. With the adoption of the small family norm by educated urban people, the need to combat genetic problems is becoming a necessity. The availability of facilities for diagnosis and management of genetic disorders and the demonstration of their impact will soon be noticed. Also, the potential for the development of molecular human genetics in India is now great. Biotechnology has been identified as a major scientific thrust area by the country and considerable resources are going into it. There are several centres in the country making use of these techniques for the control of infectious diseases and development of vaccines. Special courses in biotechnology Master's level have been started at several centres. Also, efforts to provide special biochemicals, radioisotope tracers and enzymes, etc., for molecular work are afoot, though they still remain limiting factors.

Genetics plays its most crucial and deterrent role in psychiatry. However, recent revolutionary developments in the field of psychogenetics have hardly made a discernible impact on research in India. The methods of psychiatric genetics such as family pedigree studies, twin studies, adoption studies and longitudinal studies have hardly attracted the attention of researchers in India. No one so far in this country has attempted genetic research on mental disorders in the light of developments of molecular biology, which is now the main lines of exploration in the West. The meagre amount of work that has been done relates to studies of genetic markers, and some family studies. The reasons for this situation are several. They are deeply embedded in all spheres of psychiatric research in this country, from basic orientation to finding a proper genetic research climate.

As far as genetic research in psychiatry is concerned, mental retardation has received maximum attention in India (Gupta and Sethi 1970; Sinclair 1972; Ambani et al. 1984). A recently conducted ICMR multicentre study has shown that genetic factors account for 40.3% of cases of mental retardation without a known environmental cause (unpublished observations). The magnitude and spectrum of genetic causes of mental retardation were more or less similar in different parts of India, but varied according to age groups and sources of referral at different centres participating in the study. In future in multicentric studies, such parameters also need to be controlled. Chromosomal abnormalities, particularly Down syndrome, were the most important genetic cause of mental retardation, even in a country where only 2.6% of pregnancies occur in women over 35 years of age. There is general feeling that the average age of mothers giving birth to Down's syndrome infants is lower in India, but age-related prevalence patterns have not been studied. Also, parental origin of the extra chromosome in younger women may be worth studying.

The major psychoses and some neurotic illnesses, such as obsessive compulsive disorder, where genetic factors are considered to be important, have received limited attention.

Family studies, dermatoglyphics and biochemical genetic markers are the main lines of investigation in this country whenever such studies have been carried out. Das Gupta and associates (1973), have shown that dermatoglyphics in patients with schizophrenia differ significantly from controls. In a review Balgir and Srinivasa Murthy (1982) noted that, despite the heterogeneity of schizophrenia, dermatoglyphic patterns differ significantly between schizophrenics with and without genetic loading. They have even recommended abnormal dermatoglyphics to be used as genetic marker which could differentiate schizophrenics from other disorders (Balgir et al. 1980). However, Singh and Agarwal (1980) did not find any difference between mentally retarded and schizophrenic patients. We investigated the role of genetic factors in juvenile delinquency using simple methods of sex chromatin and dermatoglyphics, but found no significant contribution of genetic factors (Agarwal et al. 1975).

In the field of major psychoses, Singh and Agarwal (1980) conducted an epidemiological, family and genetic study of primary affective disorders.

The investigators found that 90% of probands with bipolar affective illness have their first attack before reaching the age of 40, while corresponding figures for probands for unipolar illness is 72%. The morbidity risk for affective disorders in first-degree relatives was also investigated and, in the bipolar group, morbidity risks of 19.4% and 22.7% were found for parents and siblings, respectively. The estimated risk for children was found to be 10.0%. The male – female ratio of bipolar illness in probands was found to be 1 : 0.43 and, for the unipolar group, 1 : 1.6, indicating a marked excess of females suffering from unipolar illness and males from bipolar illness. The study lends further support to the contention that there are two different forms of primary affective disorders.
However, the only other report (Venkoba Rao 1974), found no such difference.

Regarding schizophrenia, family and population studies exploring genetic vulnerability have not been carried out in India. Families of schizophrenic probands have been investigated in a search for environmental factors and personality variables supposed to be related to the causation, course and outcome of schizophrenia. The only indirect work in this field has been done by one of us (Sethi et al. 1978), wherein first-degree relatives of 500 schizophrenics were investigated for the nature and frequency of psychiatric morbidity. In the available group (interviewed group) schizophrenia was the commonest illness (7.0% in first-degree relatives), followed by neurosis in 5.4% and personality disorders in 1.4%. The study did not explore the morbidity risk in parents and siblings.

Genetic studies in other psychiatric disorders have not been done in India. A small quantity of work relates to determining chromosomal abnormalities and blood groups in mental patients. Chatterjee and Basu (1981) reported a significantly high number of Barr bodies in schizophrenics, and hypothesised that during embryogenesis a questionable genetic factor caused the nondysjunction of X-chromosomes, resulting in excess Barr bodies. Datta and Jetly (1973) investigated ABO and Rhesus blood groups in 200 schizophrenics and did not find any association between ABO blood group and schizophrenia, but reported that 0 group secretors are more predisposed to schizophrenia than secretors of any other group. Singh et al. (1979) investigated ABO blood groupings in 2 000 manic-depressives and reported a bipolar group having a significantly higher frequency of blood group 0 and significantly lower frequency of blood group A, as compared with unipolar group and controls.

Certain biochemical parameters, such as platelet monoamine oxidase activity, urinary cortisol levels and platelet 5-HT uptake have been investigated. In the majority of studies relatives were not investigated, except in one from the Lucknow centre. Trivedi and associates (1988) investigated platelet monoamine oxidase activity in chronic schizophrenics, their first-degree relatives and controls, and reported significantly low enzyme activity in schizophrenics and their first-degree relatives as compared with controls.

Investigating another biochemical parameter, we have found a curious relationship between aberrations in porphyrin metabolism and psychotic disorders (Golechha et al. 1981). In addition to presentation of patients with acute intermittent porphyria with psychotic manifestations, 12.6% of patients with psychiatric disorders were found to excrete an excess amount of a porphobilinogen (PBG)-like substance in urine which differed from classical PBG in that it was extracted by butanol. A similar substance was found to be present in 2.6% of normal healthy controls. The compound remains to be identified.

The World Health Organization (WHO), through its multicentre collaborative studies, has been able to generate some data in the field of psychogenetics. The Lucknow centre has participated in these studies. In a study of variations in response to low and high doses of antidepressant drugs in different cultures carried out by WHO, it was found that response to treatment showed obvious differences in different centres (Sartorius 1981). The study indicates some differences in constitutional make-up of the patients investigated in this study (perhaps a genetic one). In another WHO multicentre study acetaldehyde dehydrogenase type-1 (ALDH-1) deficiency was found to vary across cultures. Japanese had this deficiency, but Europeans and Indians did not. ALDH deficiency is genetically inherited and absence of this deficiency is correlated with predisposition to alcoholism. In yet another ongoing WHO study, in which Lucknow is participating, hereditary and other factors are being investigated for prediction of lithium prophylactic effects. A most promising project is shortly going to be launched by WHO at its collaborating centres, aiming at development of principles of prevention of affective psychosis employing molecular and genetic approaches for identification of high risk groups. It appears that this could be a landmark study.

Psychiatric genetics is yet to develop in India in any true sense.

The impact of developments in the field of molecular genetics is yet to become apparent. There have been no molecular linkage studies in reference to psychiatric disorders and, in view of preliminary evidence that different genes may be involved in different populations in causing similar illnesses (Editorial 1988, Baron and Rainer 1988), it would be useful to ascertain the candidate genes in suitable Indian subjects.

References

Agarwal SS, Sethi N, Gupta AK, Sethi BB (1975) Buccal smear and dermatoglyphic studies in juvenile delinquency. Indian J Psychiatry 17:244–249

Agarwal SS, Lahori UC, Mehta SK, Smith DC, Bajapi PC (1979) Inheritance of Indian childhood cirrhosis. Hum Hered 29:82–89

Ambani LM, Patel ZM, Dharehwar SS, Krishnamurthy DS, Moghe MS, Mrilye VR, Gokaran VV, Peter JJ, Shah LP, Merchant SM (1984) Clinical, Biochemical and cytogenetic studies in Mental retardation. Ind J Med Res 79:384

Anonymous (1973) 'Rigveda' Part I + II. Dayanand Samstahn, New Delhi

Bala Krishnan V (1978) A preliminary study of genetic distances among some populations of the Indian subcontinent. J Hum Evol 7:67–75

Balgir RS, Srinivas Murthy R (1982) Dermatoglyphic studies in schizophrenia: a review. Ind J Psychiat 24:248–257

Balgir RS, Srinivasa Murthy R, Wig NN (1980) Manic depressive psychosis and schizophrenia: a dermatoglyphic study. Br J Psychiatry 138:558

Baron M, Rainer JD (1988) Molecular Genetic & Human Disease. Implications for modern Psychiatric Research & Practice. Brit J Psychiat 152:741–753

Basu SK (1975) Effect of consanguinity among North Indian Muslims. J Popul Res 2:57–68

Beckles GLA, Miller GJ, Kirkwood BR, Alex SD, Carson DC, Byam NTA (1986) High total and Cardiovascular disease mortality in adults of Indian descent in Trinidad, unexplained by major coronary risk factors. Lancet 1:1298–1300

Bhatia HM, Rao VR (1986) Genetic atlas of Indian tribes. Institute of Immunohaematology. ICMR, Bombay

Charak Samhita (1941) Collected and edited by Vaidya Jadavji Trikamji Acharya. 3rd Ed. Bombay, Pandurang

Chatterjee SB, Basu SK (1981) Sex chromosome aberration in schizophrenia. Indian J Psychiatry 22:142

Crow JF (1985) JBS Haldane: An appreciation. J Genetics 64:3–5

Dasgupta SN (1922) The history of Indian philosophy, vol. 1. Cambridge University Press, Cambridge

Dasgupta J, Dasgupta D, Balsubramaniyam M (1973) Dermatoglyphics in the diagnosis of schizophrenia. Indian J Psychiatry 15:104–122

Datta RN, Jetly SK (1973) Schizophrenia: its relationship with ABO and Rh blood groups. Indian J Psychiatry 15:131–135

Editorial (1988) Blue Gene. Brit Med J 297:871–872

Golecha GR, Chatterjee SB, Sethi BB, Agarwal SS (1981) Acute porphyria amongst psychiatric patients. Ind J Psychiatry 23:365–369

Gupta SC, Sethi BB (1970) Prevalence of mental retardation in Uttar Pradesh. Ind J Psychiatry 12:266

Jussawala DJ, Yeole BB, Natekar MV (1981) Histological and epidemiological features of breast cancer in different religious groups in greater Bombay. J Surg Oncol 18:269–279

Kuppuswamy B (1968) A survey of mental retardation among children enrolled in middle schools of Mysore city. Indian J Ment Retard 1:12

Liver Disease Sub-committee of ICMR (1955) Infantile cirrhosis of liver in India. Ind J Med Res 43:725–747

Majumdar DN (1961) Races & Cultures of India. Asia Publishing House, Bombay, India
Mather HM, Keen H (1985) The Southhall diabetes surveys: prevalence of known diabetes in Asians and Europeans. Br Med J 291:1981–1984
Mehra NK, Taneja V, Raizada N, Vaidya MC (1986) Distribution of HLA antigens in a sample of the North India Hindu population. Tissue Antigens 27:64–74
Mourant AE, Kopec AC, Domaniewoska Sobczak K (1976) The distribution of human blood groups and other polymorphisms. 2nd edn. Oxford University Press, London
Pitchappan RM (1988) Founder effects explain the distribution of the HLA A1-B17, but not the absence of the A1-B8 haplotypes in India. J Genet 67:101–111
Radha Rama Devi A, Appaji Rao N, Bittles AH (1987) Inbreeding and the incidence of childhood genetic disorders in Karnataka South India. J Med Genet 24:362–365
Rao PSS (1983) Religion and the intensity of inbreeding in Tamil Nadu. India Soc Biol 30:413–422
Rao, PSS, Inbaraj SG (1971) Inbreeding – effects on human reproduction in Tamil Nadu of South India. Ann Hum Genet 41:87–98
Rao PSS, Inbaraj SG (1987) Inbreeding – effects on fertility and sterility in South India. J Med Genet 24:362–365
Sanghvi LD (1966) Inbreeding in India. Eugenics Q 13:291–301
Sartorius N (1981) WHO-Coordinated collaborative studies in the effects of psychophamacological drugs in different populations. Med Probl Pharmacopsychiatry 16:83–94
Satyawati GV (ed) (1983) People of India, some genetical aspects. Publishers Indian Council of Medical Research, New Delhi, India
Sethi BB, Prakash R, Sharma M (1978) Psychiatric morbidity in first degree relatives of schizophrenia. Ind J Psychiatry 20:397–400
Sinclair S (1972) Etiological factors in Mental retardation: A study of 470 cases. Ind Pediatr 7:391
Singh G, Agarwal ML (1980) A family and genetic study of primary affective disorder. Indian J Psychiatry 22:39–50
Singh G, Agarwal ML, Sachdeva JR, Gupta AK (1979) ABO blood groups in bipolar and unipolar affective disorder. Ind J Psychiatry 22:80–83
Trivedi JK, Gupta Ashutosh K, Saxena Archana, Vishwanathan PN, Sethi BB (1988) Platelet MAO activity in first degree relatives of chronic schizophrenics. Ind J Med Res 88:360–362
Venkoba Rao R (1974) Unipolar and bipolar depression – are they different? Ind J Psychiatry 16:189–196
Verma IC (1978) High frequency of neural tube defects in North India. Lancet I:879–880
Verma IC, Mathews AR (1983) Congenital malformation in India. In: Satyawati GV (ed) People of India, some genetical aspects. Indian Council of Medical Research, New Delhi, India. ICMR, Bombay

Ethical Issues in the Application of Knowledge from Molecular Genetics to Mental Disorders

D. C. Wertz

Present State of Knowledge

At present we stand at a way station of genetic knowledge about mental disorders. We have, or soon will have, presymptomatic and prenatal tests, but no treatments. The goal of research should be treatment. Meanwhile, we are left with diagnoses. "Way station technology" is not unique in the history of medicine; diagnoses without treatments characterized most medical practice before the twentieth century. What is unique in modern genetics is the capacity to diagnose disorders many years – perhaps almost a lifetime – before onset, without being able to prevent the inevitable. This situation poses difficult ethical problems, including the following:

a) should presymptomatic tests be offered in the absence of treatment, and if so, to whom?
b) should children be tested if parents request it?
c) should a fetus be tested if parents do not want to know their own genetic status?
d) should spouses, family members at genetic risk, employers, or insurers have access to test results?
e) who should have access to, or ownership of, DNA samples?

Mental disorders pose particular problems because of the intense stigmatization that society accords their victims. Individuals at risk for these disorders have well-founded reasons for concealment from family and institutions. On the other hand, because these disorders – particularly Alzheimer's disease – are among the most financially costly for modern societies, society has a vested interest in prevention. At present, there are no proven means of preventing the onset of the most serious disorders, such as Huntington's disease (HD), in living persons; prevention must, therefore, be preconceptual or prenatal.

Limitations of Testing

The predictive value of testing is limited by the multiple etiologies present in mental disorders. With the exception of single-gene disorders such as HD, most mental disorders are probably phenotypes with many etiologies, including social, environmental, familial, and possibly viral or bacterial factors as well as genetic factors. Genetic tests do not give neat answers to patients at risk for multifactorial disorders. Usually such patients do not know what to do with the information.

What does it mean to be told, for example, that one is at 5%–10% risk for schizophrenia, on the basis of family pedigree, with no way of reducing this risk?

A further limitation of presymptomatic testing is that many genes are never expressed, or are expressed only late in life. Presymptomatic tests do not tell patients when they will develop a disease. In the case of very late-onset disorders, such as Alzheimer's, there is a good likelihood that an individual at genetic risk will not live long enough to develop the disease. Is it meaningful to learn at the age of 20 that one will develop Alzheimer's disease sometime between the ages of 70 and 100? Probably not. HD also has a variable age of onset that ranges into the 60s, and presymptomatic tests cannot tell exactly when the disorder will appear.

Finally, DNA linkage testing for some disorders is frequently impossible, usually because there are too few living family members available to provide samples. In one study of 3533 persons at risk for HD, for example, 40% lacked appropriate family structures for a linkage test (Farrer et al. 1988). Even in families with appropriate structures, tests may be uninformative or partly informative, giving intermediate risks for HD of 25%–75% rather than 1%–99%.

Given these limitations and the absence of treatment, is it ethical to offer presymptomatic or prenatal tests? Ancient wisdom said, "Seek not to know the hour of your death." Modern ethics commissions have echoed this in recommending that screening not be offered for conditions that cannot be treated (President's Commission 1983). Nevertheless, there are some arguable benefits of voluntary testing, such as planning one's life and deciding whether or not to have children.

Testing for HD can serve as a model illustrating the ethical problems inherent in presymptomatic testing for mental disorders. Although HD, as a single-gene disorder with complete penetrance, is an extreme case, it raises issues of risk and benefits, third party access to results, and stigmatization that also apply to other mental disorders.

Benefits of Testing

The major benefit of presymptomatic testing is to provide information for planning one's life and for deciding whether or not to have children. In a small number of cases, mainly those at risk for bipolar manic-depressive disorders, testing may also permit fine-tuning of medications if and when the disorder expresses itself.

Life-Planning and the Interpretation of Risk

For most people, life-plannning is the major reason for seeking testing (Mastromauro et al. 1987; Meissen and Berchek 1987; Kessler et al. 1987; Markel et al. 1987; Bird 1985; Nolan and Swenson 1988). As yet, however, there are no follow-up studies reporting what persons with positive tests actually do with the information. Whether test results affect life plans will depend upon:

a) the risk given;
b) the age of onset of the disorder;

c) the length of time between the test and the probable age of onset; and
d) the availability of support systems for people with the disorder.

With the exception of families fully informative for single-gene disorders such as HD, presymptomatic testing will likely yield probabilities rather than certainties. Most people deal poorly with probabilities. They tend to overestimate low risks, of say 2%–3%, and to underestimate high risks, say of 97%–98%. As long as a risk remains greater than zero and less then 100%, most people will not treat it as a certainty (Kahneman and Tversky 1982). People are highly variable in their interpretations of genetic risks. As long as there is no certainly, some will continue to be optimistic about high numeric risks will others will be pessimistic about low numeric risks. In general, patients interpret a given risk as lower than geneticists do. In one study of 544 genetic counseling sessions, geneticists regarded risks over 7% as "moderate" and risks over 20% as "high"; while patients regarded risks up to 15% as "low" and from 16%–50% as "moderate" (Wertz et al. 1986). *What* is risked affects the interpretation of numeric risks. If the disorder includes mental or neurological impairment, patients will interpret the risk as higher. If a family member living in the household has the disorder, patients will also interpret the risk as higher.

The form in which a risk is presented is a major factor in patients' interpretations. Most patients regard a risk of 25% as lower than a risk of 1 in 4, a risk of 20% as lower than a risk of 1 in 5, and a risk of 5% as lower than a risk of 1 in 20. This in itself presents ethical problems in counseling, because it is all too easy for a counselor to bias a patient's interpretation of a risk by choosing to present a percentage rather than a ratio, or vice versa. Presenting risks in genetic counseling does not necessarily resolve uncertainties about future plans. In a study of 836 counseling cases, almost as many (28%) left counseling as came to counseling (34%) uncertain about their reproductive plans (Wertz et al. 1984).

Added to the uncertainties inherent in numeric risk is the uncertainty about age of onset. For disorders of old age, it is questionable whether testing early in life would affect people's plans. Many would assume that they would not live long enough to develop the disorder or that a cure would be available by the time they reached old age. The longer the interval between test and probable onset, the less likely people are to use the information to make plans. If it were possible to look into the future and tell everyone, at the age of 20, the date and manner of her/his eventual death, how many would change their lifestyles and plans? Probably only those for whom the event would take place within the near future, say the next few years.

Many persons who request testing for HD fall into this category. At about the age of 35, with only a few years before possible onset, they want to be able to prepare their spouses and children for what will happen. They also wish to know whether they can afford to make major life changes, such as changing employers and thereby risking the loss of health insurance. Ironically, those whose tests are negative are the ones most likely to change their lives. They take risks – divorce, marriage, changing jobs – that they had feared to take while living in the shadow of the disease. People with positive tests tend to remain in their existing marriages and jobs; they cannot afford to risk the loss of family social support and employer-provided health insurance.

Social Planning

Marshalling social support is another putative benefit of testing; at least in theory, societies could use the results of presymptomatic tests to plan adequate financial and physical support for persons who may develop disabilities. Unfortunately, most societies have shown themselves unwilling to provide such supports. In view of past experience, there is no reason to believe that genetic testing would provide an impetus for the types of social planning that could benefit those at risk.

Reproductive Planning

Many geneticists believe that presymptomatic and prenatal testing will serve to prevent the births of children with genetic disorders. I think that we would all agree that there exists a moral obligation *not* to bring suffering into the world if we can avoid it. Some have argued that prospective parents have a moral "duty to know" their genetic status before conceiving children (Shaw 1987). In the case of late-onset disorders, however, the problem is how to balance years of useful, enjoyable life against the suffering involved in the final illness. Furthermore, there is a chance that the predicted illness will never develop because the individual has already died of some other, perhaps equally painful but nongenetic disease. In general, people may be less willing to use prenatal diagnosis and selective abortion for fetuses that will develop disorders in adulthood than they are for fetuses that will be born with a disorder. Our ongoing study of parents of children with cystic fibrosis suggests that while most would abort a fetus that would be retarded from birth or would die before the age of 5, very few would abort a fetus that would develop a severe, untreatable mental disorder at age 40. Studies suggest a profound uncertainty about aborting a fetus that would develop HD. Anywhere from 12% to 66% of persons at risk for HD say that they would use prenatal diagnosis, and 33%–71% of these would abort a fetus with the HD gene (Kessler et al. 1987; Markel et al. 1987; Mastromauro et al. 1987). At these rates, testing is unlikely to reduce the incidence of the disorder. It appears that the most likely use of prenatal diagnosis for HD may be among families who would otherwise have forgone childbearing altogether. Prenatal diagnosis therefore becomes, as it should be in democratic societies, an adjunct to individual freedom of choice rather than a means of "preventive medicine."

Therapeutic Benefits of Testing

In some instances, genetic testing allows fine-tuning of medications. In bipolar disorders where only the depression is manifest, it is useful to know whether a person is at genetic risk for manic-depression (Wexler 1989). If so, lithium is the preferred treatment, rather than antidepressants, which can precipitate the manic phase and actually make the disorder worse. A bipolar disorder can also masquerade as schizophrenia, and genetic testing could be useful in arriving at the proper prescription. Such therapeutic uses of testing are few, however.

Risks of Testing

Risks include depression, possible suicide, breaches of confidentiality, loss of job and insurance, and social stigmatization.

Psychological Sequelae of Testing

Depression always accompanies positive results of testing for HD, and may last for months. This can be treated by good follow-up counseling, continued for as long as patients need it (Meissen et al. 1988; Craufurd and Harris 1986). Usually patients overcome this initial depression and go on to cope with their situation. Although 2%–15% of patients consider themselves at risk for suicide before testing, suicide is in fact extremely rare after testing. If suicide occurs with HD, it is usually shortly after the onset of the illness itself and may either be part of the clinical syndrome or a response to loss of support (Kessler 1987). The psychological outcomes of testing itself appear to present no ethical obstacles to offering tests, provided that testing is preceded by full information and counseling and that follow-up support is provided.

Breaches of Confidentiality

The strongest ethical objection to testing arises from the very real possibility that employers and insurers will learn the results (Lamport 1987; Murray 1983; Smurl, Weaver 1987). What patients fear most is that the news will leak out and that their employers will fire them if results are positive. In nations without national health insurance, such as the United States, loss of job also means loss of health insurance, which is usually provided through employers. Insurance companies will not cover individuals at risk for chronic mental disorders. If insurers pay for the tests (few do, because there is no treatment), they usually want access to the results. Even if patients pay for tests themselves (currently about $ 4000 per family for HD), they worry that someone in the family or clinic will tell their employers. In the absence of protective legislation, this is a major reason why many people decide not to have tests.

Stigmatization

Tests for predispositions can become self-fulfilling prophecies. For example, if others know that a person is at risk for schizophrenia, they will treat her/him differently every time there is an expression of anger, and the person may indeed become schizophrenic, not for genetic reasons, but as a result of social expectations. A person at risk for Alzheimer's disease may be labeled and socially disabled at the first sign of forgetfulness, perhaps 20 or 30 years before actual neurological onset of the disease. The likelihood of stigmatization argues against testing children or young people for genetic predispositions to mental disorders. For these groups, risks outweigh benefits.

Recommendations for Offering Tests

1. All testing must be voluntary. Screening should not be considered, in accord with the general principle that it is unethical to screen for diseases that cannot be treated.
2. In view of the likelihood that for many persons the risks will outweigh the benefits, testing should *not* be encouraged. It should, however, be available for adults who want it, provided that the following conditions are met:
   a) Confidentiality can be guaranteed. Employers, insurers, schools, or other institutions should not know that a person has been tested, should not have access to results of tests, even with patients' consent, and should be legally enjoined from attempting to coerce individuals to reveal test results.
   b) The person to be tested is fully informed about the limitations of testing, including the possibility that tests may be uninformative, that they may provide mid-range probabilities that are not close to 0% or 100%, that in any case they do not provide absolute certainty, and that they do not predict age of onset.
   c) The person is mentally stable at time of testing.
   d) There is evidence that the information provided by testing would be used to prevent harm to patient, family, or prospective children.
   e) Testing is accompanied by a full pre- and post- test counseling program (see item 6).
3. Children should not be tested, even if they or their parents wish to know. Testing poses special dangers for children in their formative years, because parents and society will treat them differently if results are positive and this may precipitate psychological disorders worse than the risked disease. Although there is no clear developmental cut-off point at which testing might become appropriate, a person should have attained the age of legal majority before testing. This appears to be the best working solution, though many counselors would suggest somewhat later ages, when the person has the emotional maturity to cope with bad news. Exceptions to the rule of not testing minors would be cases of existing or intended pregnancy where the prospective parents wish to know their own genetic status or that of the fetus.
4. Individuals should have equal access to tests. Cost should not be a barrier. The only truly ethical approach is through national health insurance and nationwide testing programs, as provided, for example, in Canada. The United States approach of placing the considerable cost on individuals, to be paid out of pocket, is deplorable and is an important reason for nonutilization. If an institutional third party, including the government, pays for tests, that third party

should not have any access to test results and should not be permitted to coerce individuals into revealing results.

5. Decisions made on the basis of presymptomatic or prenatal tests should be the patient's. Counselors should not make willingness to abort affected fetuses a precondition for receiving prenatal diagnosis. Health insurers should be prohibited by law from refusing maternity coverage if an affected fetus is carried to term, and should be required to insure the child after birth.
6. Testing should take place only in the context of a *counseling program* appropriate for the disorder. For some disorders, one session may be sufficient. At the other extreme, a severe disorder such as HD may require three or four pretest counseling sessions, unlimited follow-up sessions for those with positive results, and a follow-up session for those with negative results to alleviate "survivors' guilt" (Meissen et al. 1988; Lifton 1967). For severe disorders, a single counseling session is not sufficient. Usually it takes several counseling sessions for doctors and patients to communicate their concerns. After 45–60 minutes of single-session counseling, in only 26% of cases were both patients and geneticists aware of what the other had most wanted to discuss (Wertz et al. 1988). If married, patients should be counseled together with their spouses for some of the sessions. This is especially important if children are contemplated. In a substantial minority of couples (about 40%) spouses differ from each other regarding their reproductive plans and their perceptions of the risk and burden of the disorder (Sorenson and Wertz 1986). It is therefore imperative that these differences be discussed in counseling.

Nondisclosing Tests: Special Ethical Problems

A nondisclosing test provides information about the fetus without revealing the parent's genetic status. Nondisclosing tests are of two types. In the first, DNA is not available from enough family members to provide full information about a proband, but the proband wishes to know whether a fetus will develop the disease. In these cases, a proband whose parent has HD and who is therefore at 50% risk can have the fetus tested and receive risks of roughly 1% or 49%. In other words, the fetus is either free from risk or carries the same risk as the parent. A peculiar ethical problem ensues if an at-risk fetus is carried to term. If the parent subsequently develops HD, the child is destined to develop HD and will, in effect, have been tested without giving consent. This contravenes the recommendation that children not be tested. Nevertheless, some probands who request prenatal diagnosis have no other choice, on account of their family constellations. In these situations, testing should be allowed, provided that, before testing, there is a full discussion of the possible consequences of carrying an at-risk fetus to term. Care must be taken, however, to ensure that all decisions remain the patient's.

The second type of nondisclosing test involves a proband who could learn whether he/she carries the HD gene, but does not wish to know. Instead, the proband wishes to have the fetus tested without being tested her/himself. Again, the fetus will either be virtually free of risk or will carry the same risk as the parent. Greater certainty for the fetus is not possible without testing the parent. This type of nondisclosing test is inherently unethical and should not be performed. A potential child should not be a guinea pig for a parent who does not have the courage to find out his/her own genetic status. The alternative – permitting nondisclosing tests only if parents agree in advance to abort at-risk fetuses – would be an infringement on the rights of individuals to make their own decisions.

A corollary situation arises when testing one adult would automatically disclose the genetic status of another. For example, one identical twin may wish presymptomatic testing for HD, while the other does not wish to know. It is highly unlikely that the genetic status of the tested twin could be kept a secret from the other. Demeanor or behavior would provide immediate clues about the test results. In these situations, neither twin should be tested until both have agreed to learn the results. In other words, no living person should be tested for another.

Access to Test Results: Employers and Insurers

In our 19-nation survey of 682 medical geneticists, the overwhelming majority agreed that employers and insurers should not have access to results of presymptomatic tests for HD without the patient's consent (Wertz and Fletcher 1989a and b) (Table 1). Recognizing that institutions can coerce consent by refusing employment or insurance, a substantial minority believed that these institutions should have no access at all. Their distrust is well founded. Insurance companies have made it clear that they do not intend to cover people at risk for chronic, costly disabilities such as mental disorders. Any discussion should separate health insurance from life insurance. Frequently companies sidetrack the argument by using life insurance as a specious example (e.g., by asking whether it is fair for someone to purchase $ 1 000 000 of life insurance a week before being tested for HD). The real ethical problem is health insurance, which companies usually deny to persons at risk, unless they are already covered through their employers. This means that a person who loses a job because an employer finds out about test results also irrevocably loses health insurance. People at risk dare not change jobs and dare not be honest with employers when they begin to lose functional abilities, even if they know they may be endangering others. Surgeons and firemen in the early stages of HD have continued to work after they should have retired, because they feared the loss of health insurance.

Health care is a basic right that must not be denied. It should not be confused with life insurance. There is a need for legal safeguards protecting rights to be hired, rights to continue employment as long as one remains functional, and rights to health insurance. National health insurance is the best long-term approach.

Recommendations About Employer and Insurer Access to Test Results

1. Employers should be prohibited by law from requiring presymptomatic tests for mental or neurological disorders of genetic origin either prior to hiring or as conditions of continued employment.

Table 1. Access to results of presymptomatic tests for Huntington's disease (n = 682)

Country	Percentage responding "no access to results without patient's consent" (in parentheses "no access at all")									
	Patient[a]		Spouse		Relatives at risk for HD		Employer		Life and medical insurers	
Australia	50		75[b]	(8)	67		100[b]	(67)	100[b]	(58)
Brazil	56		44	(6)	16[c]		94[b]	(31)	91[b]	(28)
Canada	67		56	(7)	65	(10)	100[b]	(54)	100[b]	(46)
Denmark	73		53	(7)	27		100[b]	(60)	100	(67)
Federal Republic of Germany	84[b]	(4)	82[b]	(7)	69	(4)	100[b]	(91)[b]	95[b]	(84)[b]
France	71	(6)	77[b]	(15)	46	(8)	100[b]	(83)[b]	100[b]	(67)
German Democratic Republic	75[b]		79[b]	(16)	65	(20)	100[b]	(89)[b]	90[b]	(85)[b]
Greece	33		17[c]		50		100[b]	(17)	83[b]	(17)
Hungary	53	(13)	67	(20)	27	(7)	93[b]	(60)	87[b]	(60)
India	30	(4)	24[c]	(4)	27	(4)	70	(35)	60	(40)
Israel	57		50		46	(8)	100[b]	(50)	100[b]	(21)
Italy	67		50	(10)	50	(10)	100[b]	(60)	100[b]	(50)
Japan	57	(8)	55	(17)	37	(14)	85[b]	(67)	88[b]	(70)
Norway	50		67		50		100[b]	(83)[b]	100[b]	(83)[b]
Sweden	71		79[b]		57		100[b]	(62)	100[b]	(48)
Switzerland	80[b]		60		80[b]		100[b]	(80)[b]	100[b]	(60)
Turkey	0[c]		0[c]		0[c]		50	(25)	75[b]	
United Kingdom	94[b]		77[b]		71		97[b]	(16)	100[b]	(19)
United States	67		65	(1)	57	(2)	98[b]	(34)	94[b]	(36)
Total	66	(2)	62	(5)	52	(4)	96[b]	(46)	93[b]	(45)
(95% confidence limits)	(61, 71)		(57, 67)		(47, 57)		(94, 98)		(90, 96)	
Total excluding United States	65	(3)	61	(7)	48	(5)	95[b]	(56)	93[b]	(52)
(95% confidence limits)	(59, 71)		(55, 67)		(42, 54)		(92, 98)		(90, 96)	

[a] Percentages are those who would tell patients only if they want to know, as opposed to informing patients against their will
[b] Strong (≥ 75%) consensus *in favor of* access only with consent
[c] Strong (≥ 75%) consensus for access *without* consent
(Wertz and Fletcher 1989a)

2. Health insurers should be prohibited by law from requiring presymptomatic tests as a condition for coverage, and prohibited from refusing coverage to persons at known genetic risk.
3. If an individual decides to be tested, employers and health insurers should be prohibited by law from access to test results, even if they paid for the test and even if the patient gives consent. If a fetus has been tested and carried to term, insurers and prospective employers should have no access to the child's test results.
4. If persons at genetic risk hold jobs involving public safety or the safety of others (e.g., persons who operate public conveyances, carry guns as part of their

duties, or perform surgery), they should be permitted to work as long as judgment and functioning remain unimpaired. Such persons should not be singled out for special tests of performance. Public safety would be better protected if employers routinely tested *all* employees at regular intervals. Persons who become disabled can be shifted into jobs where they do not endanger others. When no longer able to work, they should be retired, with full disability or retirement benefits, in accordance with the regular company benefits policy. Ideally, people should be allowed to transfer these benefits between companies, so that they will not be obliged to stay in the same job until they develop a disorder.

5. Test results should be available to government health departments and to qualified researchers for epidemiologic purposes, without identifying characteristics.
6. Life insurers may require testing as a precondition of insurance, because life insurance is not necessary for survival in daily life. In the case of late-onset disorders, people should be able to buy policies that exclude the particular disorder and perhaps also exclude suicide.

Access to Test Results: Family

One of the most difficult problems in medical genetics is whether spouses and family members at genetic risk should have access to a patient's test results without consent. There is no consensus on this issue (Table 1). Spouses and relatives have a vested interest in the information, both for reproductive planning and life-planning. They are also in the best position to provide support for a patient with long-term disabilities. Sometimes patients fear, with good reason, that spouses or family will abandon them if test results are positive, or that someone will tell their employer. Sometimes information becomes hostage to a family feud. For example, suppose the adult children seek test results from a divorced father. He refuses to tell them the results because their mother refused to allow him to visit them when they were minors. We believe that genetic information should be the common property of all family members at potential risk, not the property of individuals. Genes are shared, and family members have a moral obligation to share information that may be of use to all.

A similar situation applies to diagnoses. Presymptomatic or prenatal tests will not be used if people do not know that a disease runs in the family. It should be the moral obligation of patients with genetic disorders to tell other family members at risk about their own diagnoses. It is the moral obligation of doctors to remind patients of this. In the rare instances where a patient refuses to disclose his/her diagnosis to relatives at risk, the doctor faces a difficult dilemma between the duty to preserve patient confidentiality and the duty to warn third parties of harm (Andrews 1987). In our 19-nation survey, 32% would preserve confidentiality, 34% would tell the relatives if they asked, 24% would tell the relatives even if they did not ask, and 10% would refer the matter back to the family physician (Wertz and Fletcher 1989a) (Table 2).

Table 2. Patient confidentiality vers duties to third parties (n = 682 Geneticists). Country/Percentage who would disclose diagnosis to husband or relatives at risk for HD against patient's wishes (in parentheses percentages who would disclose even if relatives did not ask)

Australia	75[a]	(0)[b]
Brazil	91[a]	(38)
Canada	57	(32)
Denmark	87[a]	(33)
Federal Republic of Germany	74	(9)[b]
France	47	(18)[b]
German Democratic Republic	57	(43)
Greece	14[b]	(0)[b]
Hungary	47	(40)
India	48	(33)
Israel	73	(27)
Italy	82[a]	(36)
Japan	53	(16)[b]
Norway	83[a]	(50)
Sweden	48	(14)[b]
Turkey	80[a]	(60)
Switzerland	40	(20)[b]
United Kingdom	58	(32)
United States	53	(24)[b]
Total	58	(24)
(95% confidence limits)	(53, 63)	(20, 28)
Total	63	(25)
Excluding United States		
(95% confidence limits)	(57, 69)	(20, 30)

[a] Strong consensus *for* disclosure
[b] Strong consensus *against* disclosure
(Wertz and Fletcher 1989a)

Recommendations for Family Access to Test Results

1. It is the patient's moral obligation to tell relatives at risk about the diagnosis and/or results of presymptomatic tests, so that these relatives can be tested themselves. It is also a patient's moral obligation to provide blood or saliva samples so that relatives can have DNA tests.
2. It is the doctor's moral obligation to remind patients of the obligations set forth above and to continue to pressure patients until they fulfill them. "Nondirective counseling" is not appropriate in these situations. Usually patients will cooperate if repeatedly urged to do so.
3. In rare situations when patients refuse to reveal diagnoses or test results, doctors should be legally permitted to do so, taking care to provide only the relevant genetic information (not incidental findings such as false paternity). The recommendations of the President's Commission (1983) set forth the conditions under which confidentiality may be breached: "1. reasonable efforts to elicit voluntary consent to disclosure have failed; 2. there is a high probability both that harm will occur if the information is withheld and that the disclosed

information will actually be used to avert harm; 3. the harm that identifiable individuals would suffer would be serious; and 4. appropriate precautions are taken to ensure that only the genetic information needed for diagnosis and/or treatment of the disease in question is disclosed."

4. Although doctors should be legally permitted to disclose information if the four conditions listed above are fulfilled, they should not be legally required to do so unless relatives ask. Finding and disclosing information to relatives who do not ask places too much extra burden on the doctor.
5. Although genetic disorders have been compared to communicable diseases with a long latency period, such as HIV infection, it would be undesirable to require doctors to report them to public health departments, as is now done with venereal disease. Public health departments would become overburdened by trying to find and disclose information to all the relatives on large family trees. Intergenerational records of genetic diseases could become foci of ill-considered eugenic programs in the future, if such records are kept in government hands.
6. Patients have a moral obligation to inform their spouses, especially if reproduction is contemplated. Doctors have a moral obligation to remind their patients of this, and doctors should be permitted to tell spouses, without the patient's consent, if children are contemplated, according to the guidelines in item 3.
7. If family members refuse to cooperate in DNA testing, despite repeated urging, and if serious harm to others would result from this noncooperation, legal provisions may be necessary to mandate contribution of saliva, blood, or hair so that relatives can learn their own genetic status. Courts have already ordered such contributions for forensic purposes. The material contributed consists of cast-off body parts not affecting the donor's health. There is no analogy to organ donation. If contributions of DNA are mandated, care must be taken to ensure that the donor's genetic status remains confidential.

Ownership of DNA

A recent case in the United States has pointed up questions of ownership of donated blood and tissue (*John Moore* v. *The Regents of the University of California* 1988). The plaintiff argued that researchers commercially exploited products from cells that he donated with considerable time and trouble, and that he should share in the profits. The court ruled that explicit consent was required for use of cells, thereby supporting the idea that cells may be individual property. Ownership problems have already arisen with DNA that is banked for testing. Sometimes families pool their funds for DNA tests and then refuse access to those who have not contributed money. Sometimes, as with test information, banked DNA becomes hostage to family feuds or is used as a bargaining chip in divorce or custody cases. Sometimes a person refuses a specific relative access to his or her DNA because he/she believes that this relative is unable to withstand bad news.

Recommendations for Ownership of DNA

1. Ownership and disposition of DNA must be determined before blood is drawn. All patients should sign consent agreements at this time.
2. Ownership of DNA should be familial, not individual. All blood relatives should have access to stored DNA for purposes of learning their own genetic status, but not for purposes of learning the donor's status. This should be stated clearly in the consent agreement.
3. Family members should have access regardless of whether they contributed financially to the banking of the DNA.
4. DNA should be stored as long as it could be of benefit to living relatives or fetuses.
5. Attempts should be made to inform families, at regular intervals, of new developments in testing and treatments. DNA banks should keep current lists of addresses for follow-up.
6. After no relatives remain living and all attempts to contact survivors have failed, DNA may be destroyed.
7. Spouses should not have access to DNA banks without the patient's consent, but should be informed that DNA has been banked. If the couple is considering children, it is the moral obligation of the party whose DNA has been banked to tell the spouse any relevant information.
8. Insurance companies, employers, schools, and other institutional third parties should not be allowed access, even with the patient's consent.
9. Qualified researchers should have access, provided that identifying characteristics are removed.
10. Family members have a moral obligation to help each other and future generations by participating in research related to familial diseases.

Anonymous Testing for Epidemiological Purposes

Researchers and government health departments should be permitted to conduct anonymous tests on the general population in order to establish the prevalence of genetic anomalies. PCR (polymerase chain reaction) amplification has made it possible to use a single blood spot for multiple tests. Blood spots collected in screening newborns for treatable disorders could be used to provide epidemiologic information about genetic predispositions to disorders of late onset. Care must be taken to ensure that such testing remains anonymous and that results cannot be traced to individuals. Similar programs to establish prevalence of HIV infection in populations have succeeded in protecting anonymity.

Guidelines for Collaboration Between Centers

Collaboration between centers operating under different ethical guidelines poses special problems. This situation occurs frequently in cross-national or cross-cultural collaboration. Sartorius (1988) has set forth some general rules for collaboration when ethical standards differ. These include the following:

1. "The rules of the ethical review committee in the country which has the strictest regulation should be enforced for the entire collaboration network ..."
2. "The manner in which collaboration is organized should be agreed upon by all concerned and take into account culture-specific requirements and methods of work ..."
3. *All* parties should agree upon the definition of the problem to be studied and its relevance to their needs.
4. "Rules which will govern collaboration, use of data, authorship, publication of results, etc., should be discussed, agreed upon and clearly spelled out in writing before the study starts."
5. "Collaboration should not harm either of the parties." Attention should be paid to the drain that a project may place on the resources or personnel in one country and to the potential harm to other worthwhile projects. "Collaboration should not exhaust resources of a centre or team."
6. Finally, "Collaboration should leave behind a structure for future joint work."

Conclusions

Tests should be available for individuals who desire them. Such persons should be allowed to decide for themselves whether the benefits outweigh the risks, given that treatment is not yet available. Costs of testing should be borne by national health insurance or the appropriate government agency. Children below the age of legal majority should not be tested. Adults should be tested or have prenatal diagnosis only with full and proper disclosure and counseling. Legal safeguards are needed to protect individuals from employer and insurer access to test results. Patients have moral obligations to reveal their diagnoses to spouses so that relatives can be tested. Doctors have a moral obligation to remind patients of this and to provide the information to known relatives if patients will not cooperate.

In genetics, the true patient is the family, not the individual. This contravenes Western medicine's emphasis on the atomized individual. It may be necessary to transcend some individual rights in order to prevent harm to the family group. At the same time, geneticists must beware of hidden possibilities for instituting eugenic programs. Because mental disorders and disorders of aging are so costly for society, they present a special temptation for social planners.

References

Andrews LB (1987) Medical genetics: a legal frontier. American Bar Foundation, Chicago

Bird SJ (1985) Presymptomatic testing for Huntington's disease. JAMA 253 (22):3286–3291

Craufurd D, Harris R (1986) Ethics of predictive testing for Huntington's chorea: the need for more information. Br Med J 293:249–251

Farrer LA, Myers RH, Cupples LA, Conneally PM (1988) Considerations in using linkage analysis as a presymptomatic test for Huntington's disease. J Med Genet 25:577–588

Kahneman D, Tversky A (1982) The psychology of preference. Sci Am 246:160–171

Kessler S (1987) The dilemma of suicide and Huntington's disease. Am J Med Genet 26:315–317

Kessler S, Field T, Worth L, Mosbarger H (1987) Attitudes of persons at risk for Huntington's disease toward predictive testing. Am J Med Genet 26:259–270

Lamport AT (1987) Presymptomatic testing for Huntington's chorea: ethical and legal issues. Am J Med Genet 26:307–314

Lifton RJ (1967) Death in life: survivors of Hiroshima. Random House, New York

Markel DS, Young AB, Penney JB (1987) At-risk persons' attitudes toward presymptomatic and prenatal testing of Huntington's disease in Michigan. Am J Med Genet 26:295–305

Mastromauro C, Myers RH, Berkman B (1987) Attitudes toward presymptomatic testing in Huntington's disease. Am J Med Genet 26:271–282

Meissen GJ, Berchek RL (1987) Intended use of predictive testing by those at risk for Huntington's disease. Am J Med Genet 26:283–293

Meissen GJ, Myers RH, Mastromauro CA, Koroshetz WJ, Klinger KW, Farrer LA, Watkins PA, Gusella JF, Bird ED, Martin JB (1988) Predictive testing for Huntington's disease with use of a linked DNA marker. N Engl J Med 318:535–542

Murray TH (1983) Warning: screening workers for genetic risk. Hastings Center Rep 13:5–8

Nolan K, Swenson S (1988) New tools, new dilemmas: genetic frontiers. Hastings Center Rep Oct/Nov:40–46

President's Commission for the Study of Ethical Problems in Medicine and Biomedical and Behavioral Research (1983) Screening and counseling for genetic conditions. US Government Printing Office, Washington

Sartorius N (1988) Cross-cultural and international collaboration in mental health research and action: experience from the mental health programme of the World Health Organization. Acta Psychiatr Scand 78 [344, Suppl]:71–74

Shaw MW (1987) Testing for the Huntington gene: a right to know, a right not to know, or a duty to know. Am J Med Genet 26:243–246

Smurl JF, Weaver DD (1987) Presymptomatic testing for Huntington's chorea: guidelines for moral and social accountability. Am J Med Genet 26:247–257

Sorenson JR, Wertz DC (1986) Couple agreement before and after genetic counseling. Am J Med Genet 25:549–555

Wertz DC, Fletcher JC (1989a) Ethics and human genetics: a cross-cultural perspective. Springer, Berlin Heidelberg New York

Wertz DC, Fletcher JC (1989b) An international survey of attitudes of medical geneticists toward mass screening and access to results. Public Health Rep 104(1):35–44

Wertz DC, Sorenson JR, Heeren TC (1984) Genetic counseling and reproductive uncertainty. Am J Med Genet 18:79–88

Wertz DC, Sorenson JR, Heeren TC (1986) Clients' interpretations of risks provided in genetic counseling. Am J Hum Genet 39:253–264

Wertz DC, Sorenson JR, Heeren TC (1988) Communication in health professional-lay encounters: how often does each party know what the other wants to discuss? In: Ruben BD (ed) Information and behavior 2. Transaction Books, New Brunswick NJ, pp 329–342

Wexler NS (1989) The oracle of DNA. In: Rowland LP, Wood DS, Schon EA, DiMauro S (eds) Molecular genetics in diseases of brain, nerve, and muscle. Oxford University Press, New York, pp 429–442

The Potential and the Pitfalls of Molecular Genetics for Psychiatry: An Overview

R. M. Murray and *M. Gill*

Introduction

The successful application of molecular genetic techniques to psychiatric disorders is likely to require the expertise of at least three separate types of researcher:
a) clinicians familiar with the use of operational definitions of psychiatric illness,
b) molecular biologists knowledgeable about neurobiology, and
c) statistical geneticists sufficiently versatile to be able not only to perform various types of analyses on complex diseases but also to place the results in the appropriate epidemiological context.

The conference on which this book is based brought together representatives of each of these groups to review the rapidly changing field of psychiatric genetics and to plan how the World Health Organisation (WHO) could facilitate further developments. This chapter highlights some of the main themes which emerged.

Can Standard "Reverse Genetic" Techniques be Applied?

Much of the meeting focused on the extent to which psychiatric disorders may prove amenable to molecular genetic techniques in general and "reverse genetics" in particular. Psychiatric disorders are, or at present appear to be, multifactorial, while the early successes of molecular genetics concerned fully penetrant single-gene disorders. This, however, should not be an insuperable hurdle, as molecular techniques are beginning to resolve other polygenic conditions such as coronary heart disease and diabetes. More problematic is the question of whether disorders such as schizophrenia or manic-depressive psychosis are discrete entities with a single major cause or at least a common pathogenic pathway. No clear answer is yet available, but much contemporary opinion regards the major psychoses as clinical syndromes which will ultimately be broken down into their constituent parts (Murray et al. 1985). If this is true, the geneticist is faced with the equivalent of attempting to unravel the molecular basis of renal failure rather than the easier task of resolving the genetics of polycystic kidney disease.

Fortunately, there is no doubt that molecular genetic techniques are applicable to disorders of the central nervous system. Huntington's disease was the first condition for which the responsible gene was localised, and now the genes for numerous other neurological disorders have been approximately located in a similar way

(Martin 1987). Unfortunately, most conditions described by Martin are not convincing models for psychiatric disorders because:

a) they are single-gene disorders,
b) although they may have behavioural consequences they are not primarily behavioural disorders, and
c) although diagnostic difficulties do exist, in general the disease phenotype is much more characteristic.

Alzheimer's disease has emerged as a more appropriate model. Firstly, the manifestations are primarly psychological. Secondly, it does not have a single cause and indeed, until recently, few authorities believed that heredity was of much importance. Thirdly, it has been subject to many of the same disputes concerning its status as a discrete entity and the vagueness of its boundaries as other psychiatric disorders. Nevertheless, two separate groups (St. George-Hyslop et al. 1987; Goate et al. 1989) have reported linkage between early-onset familial Alzheimer's disease and a locus on the long arm of chromosome 21. It is of course true that in contrast to the major functional psychoses, Alzheimer's disease has

a) a more uniform course and outcome and
b) a characteristic neuropathology.

However, now that a linkage has been confirmed for familial Alzheimer's disease, perhaps the same general strategy may be applicable to other psychiatric disorders.

The Epidemiological Context

Linkage studies, by their nature, concentrate on multiply affected pedigrees in the belief that such pedigrees are likely to result from the operation of a single mutant gene. In their chapter in this volume, McGue and Gottesman point out, however, that one cannot assume that such loaded pedigrees are necessarily segregating for a major gene, since their existence would also be expected under a multifactorial polygenic model. Furthermore, even if pedigrees are found in which linkage studies do indicate the operation of a single major gene, it is important to remember that such a sampling strategy selects for atypical cases. Goldstein et al. (1989) found that, when familial schizophrenia is defined on the basis of the disorder occurring in one or more first-degree relatives, only 8% of some 322 schizophrenic probands qualified.

In addition, our own experience is that fewer than one in ten of all familial cases turns out to have come from a suitable multiply affected family willing to cooperate in molecular genetic studies. Thus, linkage studies of schizophrenia are likely to be sampling less than the extreme 1% of all cases. The rarity of such families in practice is in accord with the prediction of McGue and Gottesman's modelling. They calculate that for all the likely models of transmission, a maximum of four schizophrenic probands out of approximately 1300 are likely to come from nuclear families in which there are four or more affected members. If linkage is found in such families, with a single highly penetrant gene, as appears indicated in the report of Sherrington et al. (1988), in theory it may be confined to similar multiplex families.

Molecular geneticists point out that to discover the cause of at least one, albeit rare, form of schizophrenia would represent a major step forward, and that this knowledge could indicate where to look in the wider context. Alternatively, a mutant gene implicated in highly familial cases could, in most circumstances, have a much lower penetrance and thus explain apparently sporadic cases. McGue and Gottesman's calculations indicate that a single-gene model does not adequately account for either the twin or dual mating data, although a single major gene against a polygenic background could. If true, these calculations have important implications for the likelihood of finding linkage. However, the very sophistication of the complex genetic models being proposed makes them very difficult to disprove. They contrast in principle with the reductionist approach of molecular biology, where real date, even if negative, can provide a stimulus to tackle what initially may appear an unsurmountable task.

It is not sensible to expect to resolve these issues in the abstract. If the pessimistic prognostications of Sturt and McGuffin (1985) had been taken to their logical conclusion, the endeavour to apply molecular techniques to psychiatric disorders would probably not have commenced. The answers will have to await experimental data.

Failure of Replication

It is remarkable, in light of the difficulties discussed above, that there have been so many significantly positive results from linkage experiments to data. It is clear, however, that failure to replicate claims of linkage in a wider range of pedigrees is more common in psychiatric than medical genetics. Indeed, the initial reports of linkage of manic-depression and schizophrenia to markers on chromosome 11 and 5, respectively, were accompanied by negative reports (Hodgkinson et al. 1987, Kennedy et al. 1988). These were taken to imply genetic heterogeneity rather than as lack of support for the original claim (Lander 1988; Byerley et al. 1989). This may yet be so, but there are alternative explanations including the possibility that there are flaws in the principles underlying the application of the LOD score method or in the manner in which it has been employed, which allows the conventional level of significance for linkage in a monogenic medical disorder to be reached in the more complex psychiatric conditions without conveying the same level of certainty.

In psychiatric disorders, linkage studies cannot be undertaken without first making assumptions concerning not only the definition of the phenotypes but also the mode of transmission and other genetic parameters, such as disease frequency and penetrance of the abnormal genotype. In this volume Bertelsen reviews the problems involved in defining the phenotype. In her chapter Clerget-Darpoux notes that the LOD score method is sensitive to the use of the wrong genetic parameters, such as allele frequencies and penetrance values, but concludes that such erroneous specifications should decrease the power to detect linkage. Thus, such errors should not produce false-positive results but could account for failure to replicate genuine findings.

False-negative findings may yet turn out to be more problematic than false positives. Clerget-Darpoux points out that it is very tempting for researchers to perform LOD score analyses using different genetic models, different parameter values, and different diganostic models, and thus maximise the LOD score. This may well be a legitimate exercise given that the parameters are unknown in the first place, but extreme caution must be exercised if bias is to be avoided. Positive findings of linkage need to be checked in a number of ways. Firstly, they need to be replicated in the true sense; this involves an assessment by independent researchers using the same basic data concerning all factors, including diagnosis of the phenotypes, ascertainment of the genotypes at the relevant marker loci, and the statistical analysis. Secondly, the relevant markers need to be examined in other appropriate pedigrees, using the same diagnostic models and genetic parameters. Thirdly, the original data need to be expanded. This can be achieved by extending the pedigrees as far as is possible, by rendering existing members more informative for the relevant markers, or by examining the segregation of other, more informative markers which are closely linked to existing markers. If the linkage is true, all these manipulations will lead to an increase in the LOD score.

Further investigation of the Amish pedigree reported by Egeland et al. (1987) had had the opposite effect on the LOD score. Firstly, additional affected individuals were found within the core pedigree who were obligate recombinants with either marker, and this lowered the LOD score. Secondly, a lateral extension, which appeared to have a different genetic source of the disorder, showed no linkage between the 11p15 markers and affective disorder (Kelsoe et al. 1989). Clearly, a LOD score of 3 should not be taken as other than suggestive evidence of the existence of a mutant gene. It must be remembered that such LOD scores can occur by chance, and, for some as yet unknown reason, this may occur more frequently when the LOD score method is applied to complex disorders. Although chance occurrences of false positives are implicit in the LOD score method, it may be necessary to make some correction to the significance level, taking into account the number of markers tested, as has been suggested by Edwards and Watt (1989).

The Implications of Confirmed Linkage

Once a linkage has been firmly established for one of the major psychiatric disorders (or a subset of it, as in Alzheimer's disease), the full range of molecular techniques for moving from linkage to the gene can be brought to bear. In diseases such as cystic fibrosis, genetic mapping using new markers has been valuable in further limiting the possible site of the disease gene. This involves examining these markers for crossovers in linked pedigrees between the disease phenotype and the marker locus. If the new marker shows no crossover where one was seen with the existing marker, this marker is likely to be nearer the disease gene. However, as Williamson and Goate point out in this volume, the likely existence of genetic heterogeneity, incomplete penetrance, and diagnostic ambiguity will reduce the power of such genetic mapping. As a result, the isolation of the mutant genes in psychiatric disorders will rely more on the use of physical techniques to isolate and map markers in the vicinity of the disease gene. Such techniques include pulsed-field electrophoresis – a method of examining very large fragments – and yeast artificial chromosomes (YACs) – a method of cloning such large fragments. Although the use of these tools can order a large set of DNA markers on a map, it is difficult to see how the disease gene can be placed on this map without using genetic mapping. This is likely to require many more informative meioses than are conceivable in the psychiatric disorders. The use of physical mapping techniques in Huntington's disease is described by Bates and Lehrach in their chapter, but even in this relatively uncomplicated disorder, with a great many meioses available for study, the actual isolation of the gene has proved a lengthy, and as yet unrealised, process.

A successful confirmation of linkage would, of course, have important consequences. Firstly, it would clearly establish the existence of a single gene and its mode of transmission in at least a subset of the disorder; secondly it would have implications for psychiatric nosology. It seems unlikely that our present-day system of psychiatric classification bears any close relationship to aetiological reality. Hopefully, linkage studies will begin the process of establishing the boundaries of disorders defined on aetiological rather than phenomenological grounds (Mullan and Murray 1989). It may be that a single genetic defect can express itself in a variety of phenotypes; alternatively, different mutations at a single locus may account for the variable phenotypes seen, for example, in schizophrenia. Conversely, abnormalities at different loci may cause the same clinical presentation. It may be that such differences will have clinical consequences. For example, chromosome 21 linked Alzheimer's disease appears to be associated with early onset and poor outcome (Hardy, personal communication). Similarly, in this volume Mendlewicz suggests that X-linked manic depression may be associated with early presentation, lack of clinical response, and poor outcome.

Molecular Biology and Neuroscience

Hitherto, this discussion has concentrated on linkage studies using anonymous DNA markers, in a reverse genetics approach. The approach adopted by Bloom et al. (this volume) is the more fundamental one of trying to identify the mRNA species (and hence the genes) which determine the characteristic structural and functional properties of the cerebral cortex. The brain expresses some 30 000 or more genes, of which probably some 30% are relatively brain specific. How does the molecular biologist determine which may be fundamental to neuropsychiatric dysfunction? Bloom et al. are concentrating on three areas; the visual, motor and prefrontal cortex, of which the latter will probably be of most import to psychiatrists. This is clearly a very long term project, but interesting examples are already being found: for example, the hypocerebellar mouse mutant 'jimpy' whose defective myelination during development arises from a missing segment in a proteolipid gene. Further work reported by Bloom et al. concerns the elucidation of those hypothalamic brain cells which express mRNA for the neurohormone oxytocin. There are, of course, sex differences in such expression and considerable changes at puberty; the latter may be of relevance to the fact that the major psychoses frequently have their onset in late adolescence and early adult life. Similarly the genetic control of myelination during development is of great interest to those who postulate that this process may be involved in the manifestation of schizophrenic symptoms (Weinberger 1987; Murray et al. 1988).

It is reasonable to postulate that the differences in neuronal architecture, circuitry and signalling in different brain regions are due to the effects, either singly or in combination, of relatively rare brain mRNAs. It is therefore logical to study tissue from those brain areas thought to be involved in different disorders, for example, the parahippocampal gyrus in schizophrenia. We should, of course, recall that in this particular psychosis, structural anomalies appear to arise very early in development (Murray et al. 1988). It will therefore be important to examine mRNA isolated from tissues at various times during development as well as in adult life.

There are other approaches which are neither 'top down', as in linkage analyses, nor 'bottom up', as discussed in the preceding paragraphs. One such approach involves the intensive study of 'candidate genes'. Neurotransmitter-related genes are obvious candidate genes, and association studies have already begun examining, for example, tyrosine hydroxylase (Mallet 1989). Similar studies are being carried out using the dopamine D_2 receptor gene in psychosis, and alcohol dehydrogenase and aldehyde dehydrogenase genes in families with several alcoholic members.

Another such approach concerns the examination of pedigrees in which disorder appears to co-segregate with a chromosomal translocation or deletion. Already the report of Bassett et al. (1988) has stimulated great interest in chromosome 5. Similarly, Holland et al. and Blackwood et al. in Great Britain and Potkin in California are studying families in which balanced translocations involve as one of their breakpoints chromosome 11p, which appears to co-segregate with psychosis, thus rendering this a candidate region. In contrast to a region of trisomy, a balanced translocation my pinpoint the exact site of the gene, rendered mutant by disruption due to one or other translocation breakpoints.

The Role of the WHO

What can the WHO do to further research into the genetics of psychiatric disorders? Firstly, it can continue to sponsor workshops such as that reported in this volume, at which researchers from varying backgrounds can resolve their differences in a productive manner. For example, at this workshop, it has become clear that molecular biologists tend to hold robustly reductionist views, confident that single genes of major effect will be located not only for Alzheimer's disease but also in the functional psychoses, alcoholism, and possibly some neurotic disorders. At the other extreme are those such as Gottesman who believe that psychiatric disorders are generally multifactorial, and that, for instance, it is unrealistic to expect that more than 5% of all schizophrenia will be attributable to the sole action of a major gene.

Nevertheless, all participants acknowledged that spectacular progress had been made in many neurological disorders, and one psychiatric condition (Alzheimer's disease). It was also agreed that premature claims of linkage will retard progress; this caution is likely to have been increased by the rise and subsequent fall of the LOD score in the affective disorder study among the Amish (Kelsoe et al. 1989).

Productive discussions also took place concerning the size and number of pedigrees necessary to demonstrate linkage in the face of varying degrees of genetic heterogeneity. There was also considerable interest in non-parametric alternative to the LOD score method, such as the use of affected sib pairs. Affected sib pairs are easier to come by than multigeneration families, and the method does not depend on assumptions about the mode of transmission. On the other hand, it loses information from the unaffected members and is ineffective in the presence of all but relative homogeneity. As noted above, multiply affected families are relatively rare, and it is expensive to carefully obtain the necessary clinical information; there is much, therefore, to be gained through different research groups exchanging DNA from well investigated pedigrees. A related function is to encourage the collection of clinical data in a comprehensive and systematic manner; in this way not only will studies be comparable, but it should also be possible to pool data. The likely heterogeneity of psychiatric disorders means that it may be necessary to screen the whole genome in a very large number of families and to analyse the data as one. Facilitating such collaboration will be a valuable function for the WHO, perhaps in cooperation with other international agencies such as the European Science Foundation and the National Institutes of Health in the United States. The WHO has a distinguished history of involvement in the cross-cultural collection of data. This expertise should be put to good use not only in ensuring a high standard of clinical description but also in widening the scope of much genetic investigation.

The current approaches could profitably be broadened in three ways. The first is by combining molecular genetic studies with studies of other biological markers known to be associated with the disease under scrutiny. For example, in schizophrenia we need to enquire into whether any chromosome 5 linked forms are associated with abnormalities of event-related potentials (P300) or of smooth-pursuit eye movements. Indeed as Lander (1988) notes, instead of attempting to map schizophrenia per se, it may be more fruitful to map the genetic basis for some biological abnormality associated with it. Secondly, nearly all family, twin, and adoption studies of psychiatric disorders have been carried out in Western Europe or North America. Consequently, we do not know whether psychiatric disorders as seen in the developing world are under a similar degree of genetic influence. The WHO, with its extensive connections in developing countries, could usefully promote studies to address this issue. Thirdly, it is important to recall that genetic studies can also tell us something concering the influence of the environment. Therefore, studies should address the question of what protects individuals who carry susceptibility gene(s) but remain well. Similarly, we need to know the relationship between environmental pathogenic factors such as adverse life events and genetic predisposition, again an area in which the expertise of the WHO is of considerable value.

Finally, molecular genetic studies are already posing difficult questions for society. On the one hand, they offer a huge potential for improving the prevention and treatment of mental diseases. On the other, individuals and society will be increasingly confronted with difficult dilemmas. Some of these are reviewed by Wertz (this volume) and by Pelosi and David (1990). This is a field in which opinions tend to become polarised. The WHO may well be able to play an important moderating role here, not only within the scientific community but also in the wider public world, through its relationships with governments and health educators in different cultures.

References

Bassett AS, Jones BD, McGillivray BC, Pantzar JT (1988) Partial trisomy chromosome 5 cosegregating with schizophrenia. Lancet I:799–801

Byerley W, Mellon C, O'Connell PO, Lalouel JM Nakamura Y, Leppert M, White R (1989) Mapping genes for manic-depression and schizophrenia with DNA markers. Trends Neurosci 12:46–48

Edwards JH, Watt DC (1989) Caution in locating the gene(s) for affective disorder. Psychol Med 19:273–275

Egeland JA, Gerhard DS, Pauls DL, Sussex JN, Kidd KK, Allen CR, Hostetter AM, Housman DE (1987) Bipolar affective disorders linked to DNA markers on chromosome 11. Nature 325:783–787

Goate AM, Haynes AR, Owen MJ, Jarrall M, James LA, Lai LY-C, Mullan MJ, Roques P, Rosser MN, Williamson R, Hardy JA (1989) Predisposing locus to Alzheimer's disease on chromosome 21. Lancet I:352–355

Goldstein BJ, Santangelo SL, Simpson JC, Tsuang MT (1989) The role of gender in identifying subtypes of schizophrenia. Schizophr Bull (in press)

Hodgkinson S, Sherrington R, Gurling H, Marchbanks R, Reeders S, Mallet J, McInnis M, Petursson H, Brynjolfsson J (1987) Molecular genetic evidence for heterogeneity in manic depression. Nature 325:805–806

Kelsoe JR, Ginns EI, Egeland JA, Goldstein AM, Bale SJ, Pauls DL, Long RT, Conte G, Gerhard DS, Houseman DE, Paul SM (1989) Reevaluation of the linkage relationship between chromosome 11p loci and the gene for bipolar affective disorder in the old order Amish. Nature 342:238–242

Kennedy JL, Giuffra LA, Moises HW, Cavalli-Sforza LL, Pakstis AJ, Kidd JR, Castiglione C, Sjøogren B, Wetterberg L, Kidd KK (1988) Evidence against linkage of schizophrenia to markers on chromosome 5 in a northern Swedish pedigree. Nature 336:167–169

Lander ES (1988) Splitting schizophrenia. Nature 336:105–106

Martin JB (1987) Molecular genetics: application to the clinical neurosciences. Science 238:765–772

Mullan M and Murray RM (1989) The impact of molecular genetics on our undertanding of the psychoses. Br J Psychiatry 154:591–595

Murray RM, Lewis SW, Reveley AM (1985) Towards an aetiological classification of schizophrenia. Lancet I:1023–1026

Murray RM, Lewis SW, Owen MJ, Foerster A (1988) The neurodevelopmental origins of dementia praecox. In: Bebbington P, McGuffin P (eds) Schizophrenia: the major issues. Heinman, London, pp 90–107

Pelosi AJ, David AS (1990) Ethical implications of the new genetics for psychiatry. Int Rev Psychiatry (in press)

Sherrington R, Brynjolfsson J, Petursson H, Potter M, Dudleston K, Barraclough B, Wasmuth J, Dobbs M, Gurling H (1988) Localization of a susceptibility locus for schizophrenia on chromosome 5. Nature 336:164–167

St. George-Hyslop PH, Tanzi RE, Polinsky RJ, Haines JL, Nee L, Watkins PC, Meyers RH, Feldman RG, Pollen D, Drachman D, Growdon J, Bruni A, Foncin J-F, Salmon G, Fromhelt

P, Amaducci L, Sorgi S, Placentini S, Stewaqrt GD, Hobbs W, Conneally PM, Gusella JF (1987) The genetic defect causing familial Alzheimer's disease maps on chromosome 21. Science 235:885–890
Sturt E, McGuffin P (1985) Can linkage and marker association resolve the genetic aetiology of psychiatric disorders? Review and argument. Psychol Med 15:455–462
Weinberger DR (1987) Implications of normal brain development for the pathogenesis of schizophrenia. Arch Gen Psychiatry 44:660–669

Subject Index

GPSR Compliance
The European Union's (EU) General Product Safety Regulation (GPSR) is a set of rules that requires consumer products to be safe and our obligations to ensure this.

If you have any concerns about our products, you can contact us on

ProductSafety@springernature.com

In case Publisher is established outside the EU, the EU authorized representative is:

Springer Nature Customer Service Center GmbH
Europaplatz 3
69115 Heidelberg, Germany

www.ingramcontent.com/pod-product-compliance
Ingram Content Group UK Ltd.
Pitfield, Milton Keynes, MK11 3LW, UK
UKHW051353110926
15112UKWH00020B/168
* 9 7 8 3 6 6 2 0 7 4 2 2 0 *